GETTING iNTO NURSiNG

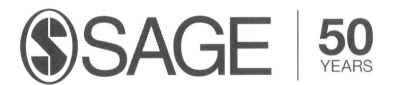

SAGE was founded in 1965 by Sara Miller McCune to support the dissemination of usable knowledge by publishing innovative and high-quality research and teaching content. Today, we publish more than 750 journals, including those of more than 300 learned societies, more than 800 new books per year, and a growing range of library products including archives, data, case studies, reports, conference highlights, and video. SAGE remains majority-owned by our founder, and after Sara's lifetime will become owned by a charitable trust that secures our continued independence.

Los Angeles | London | Washington DC | New Delhi | Singapore

GETTING INTO NURSING

2ND EDITION

KAREN ELCOCK

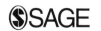

Los Angeles | London | New Delhi
Singapore | Washington DC | Boston

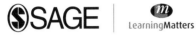

Learning Matters
An imprint of SAGE Publications Ltd
1 Oliver's Yard
55 City Road
London EC1Y 1SP

SAGE Publications Inc.
2455 Teller Road
Thousand Oaks, California 91320

SAGE Publications India Pvt Ltd
B 1/I 1 Mohan Cooperative Industrial Area
Mathura Road
New Delhi 110 044

SAGE Publications Asia-Pacific Pte Ltd
3 Church Street
#10–04 Samsung Hub
Singapore 049483

Editor: Alex Clabburn
Development editor: Caroline Sheldrick
Production controller: Chris Marke
Project management: Swales & Willis Ltd,
    Exeter, Devon
Marketing manager: Camille Richmond
Cover design: Wendy Scott
Typeset by: C&M Digitals (P) Ltd, Chennai, India
Printed by: CPI Group (UK) Ltd, Croydon, CR0 4YY

Library of Congress Control Number: 2015930290

British Library Cataloguing in Publication Data

A catalogue record for this book is available from
the British Library

ISBN 978-1-4739-0260-2
ISBN 978-1-4739-0261-9 (pbk)

At SAGE we take sustainability seriously. Most of our products are printed in the UK using FSC papers and boards.
When we print overseas we ensure sustainable papers are used as measured by the Egmont grading system.
We undertake an annual audit to monitor our sustainability.

Contents

Transforming Nursing Practice is a series tailor-made for pre-registration student nurses. Each book in the series is:

- Affordable
- Mapped to the NMC Standards and Essential Skills Clusters
- Full of active learning features
- Focused on applying theory to practice

Each book addresses a core topic and they have been carefully developed to be simple to use, quick to read and written in clear language.

> An invaluable series of books that explicitly relates to the NMC standards. Each book cover a different topic that students need to explore in order to develop into a qualified nurse... I would recommend this series to all Pre-Registration nursing students whatever their field or year of study
>
> **Linda Robson**
> **Senior Lecturer, Edge Hill University**
>
> The set of books is an excellent resource for students. The series is small, easily portable and valuable. I use the whole set on a regular basis.
>
> **Fiona Davies**
> **Senior Nurse Lecturer, University of Derby**
>
> I recommend the SAGE/Learning Matters series to all my students as they are relevant and concise. Please keep up the good work.
>
> **Thomas Beary**
> **Senior Lecturer in Mental Health Nursing, University of Hertfordshire**

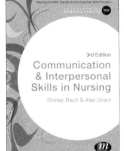

3rd Edition
Communication & Interpersonal Skills in Nursing
Shirley Bach & Alec Grant

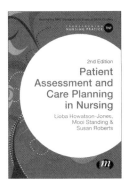

2nd Edition
Patient Assessment and Care Planning in Nursing
Lioba Howatson-Jones, Mooi Standing & Susan Roberts

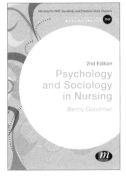

2nd Edition
Psychology and Sociology in Nursing
Benny Goodman

ABOUT THE SERIES EDITORS

Professor Shirley Bach is Head of the School of Health Sciences at the University of Brighton and responsible for the core knowledge titles. Previously she was head of post-graduate studies and has developed curriculum for undergraduate and pre-registration courses in a variety of subject domains.

Dr Mooi Standing is an Independent Academic Consultant (UK and International) and responsible for the personal and professional learning skills titles. She is an accredited NMC Quality Assurance Reviewer of educational programmes and a Professional Regulator Panellist on the NMC Practice Committee.

Sandra Walker is Senior Teaching Fellow in Mental Health at the University of Southampton and responsible for the mental health nursing titles. She is a Qualified Mental Health Nurse with a wide range of clinical experience spanning more than 20 years.

CORE KNOWLEDGE TITLES:

Becoming a Registered Nurse: Making the Transition to Practice

Communication and Interpersonal Skills in Nursing (3rd Ed)

Contexts of Contemporary Nursing (2nd Ed)

Getting into Nursing (2nd Ed)

Health Promotion and Public Health for Nursing Students (2nd Ed)

Introduction to Medicines Management in Nursing

Law and Professional Issues in Nursing (3rd Ed)

Leadership, Management and Team Working in Nursing (2nd Ed)

Learning Skills for Nursing Students

Medicines Management in Children's Nursing

Nursing and Collaborative Practice (2nd Ed)

Nursing and Mental Health Care

Nursing in Partnership with Patients and Carers

Passing Calculations Tests for Nursing Students (3rd Ed)

Palliative and End of Life Care in Nursing

Patient Assessment and Care Planning in Nursing (2nd Ed)

Patient and Carer Participation in Nursing

Patient Safety and Managing Risk in Nursing

Psychology and Sociology in Nursing (2nd Ed)

Successful Practice Learning for Nursing Students (2nd Ed)

Understanding Ethics in Nursing Practice

Using Health Policy in Nursing

What is Nursing? Exploring Theory and Practice (3rd Ed)

PERSONAL AND PROFESSIONAL LEARNING SKILLS TITLES:

Clinical Judgement and Decision Making for Nursing Students (2nd Ed)

Critical Thinking and Writing for Nursing Students (2nd Ed)

Evidence-based Practice in Nursing (2nd Ed)

Information Skills for Nursing Students

Reflective Practice in Nursing (2nd Ed)

Succeeding in Essays, Exams & OSCEs for Nursing Students

Succeeding in Literature Reviews and Research Project Plans for Nursing Students (2nd Ed)

Successful Professional Portfolios for Nursing Students (2nd Ed)

Understanding Research for Nursing Students (2nd Ed)

MENTAL HEALTH NURSING TITLES:

Assessment and Decision Making in Mental Health Nursing

Engagement and Therapeutic Communication in Mental Health Nursing

Medicines Management in Mental Health Nursing

Mental Health Law in Nursing

Physical Healthcare and Promotion in Mental Health Nursing

Psychosocial Interventions in Mental Health Nursing

ADULT NURSING TITLES:

Acute and Critical Care in Adult Nursing

Caring for Older People in Nursing

Medicines Management in Adult Nursing

Nursing Adults with Long Term Conditions

Safeguarding Adults in Nursing Practice

Dementia Care in Nursing

You can find more information on each of these titles and our other learning resources at **www.sagepub.co.uk**. Many of these titles are also available in various e-book formats, please visit our website for more information.

About the authors

Karen Elcock is Head of Programmes, Pre-registration Nursing and Deputy Head of School at Kingston University and St George's, University of London, one of the early implementers of the new degree programme for nursing. She has taught and led on pre-registration nursing programmes for over 20 years and has a particular interest in how student nurses learn in practice settings, which make up 50% of pre-registration nursing programmes.

The chapter contributors are also all current or former staff from Kingston University and St George's, University of London.

Mary Brady is Senior Lecturer and Field Lead for Child Health.

Rosi Castle is Senior Lecturer and Field Lead for Adult Nursing.

Maggie Davenport is Principal Lecturer and Course Director for the Postgraduate Diploma in Nursing programme.

Beattie Dray is a former Principal Lecturer in Recruitment and Retention and now an independent Consultant.

Sue Fergy is Clinical Lead, Multiprofessional Faculty Development (London).

Mandy Gough is Academic Skills Centre Co-ordinator.

Martyn Keen is Senior Lecturer and Field Lead for Mental Health.

Andrew Perkins is Senior Lecturer Nursing and Academic Skills.

Penny Smith is Senior Lecturer – Learning Disability Nursing.

Kim Tolley is Regional Liaison Adviser, General Medical Council

Foreword

It might seem improbable that there needs to be a text on guiding potential applicants to nursing. The process of going through UCAS and submitting personal statements is usually supported by sound advice from college tutors and is not an unfamiliar activity, as the numbers of young adults attending university is rising year on year. A nursing qualification is now only achieved through a full university degree. The perception is that only a few highly motivated individuals wish to go into nursing, yet the numbers of applicants to nursing degree courses are increasing. Consequently, the competition for places is escalating and the application process is being carefully refined to choose only the most suitable and academically able candidates.

The authors have shared their considerable experience of selecting recruits into nursing and have a significant understanding of the attributes and characteristics applicants need to demonstrate throughout the selection process. It is important to understand that the selection process has many facets because universities are looking for several different qualities. They are choosing applicants who can undertake a demanding three-year period of study *and* who are also suitable to enter into a profession that requires high levels of personal characteristics such as integrity and compassion. Interview processes are now firmly anchored in methods that are based upon values and attitudes.

In this text you will find an explanation of contemporary nursing, bearing in mind the recent emphasis highlighted in government reports on nursing practice with caring and compassion being essential elements of nursing, the different fields of nursing and specialties of nursing practice. This helps you to prepare for questions on the role of nursing. There are also practical chapters on entry requirements, what is expected of applicants, the various entrance tests (e.g. literacy and numeracy that all candidates have to undertake) and the various selection methods used at interview to identify your personal characteristics and suitability.

In keeping with the style of the Transforming Nursing Practice series, there are many activities and case studies to illustrate the topics being discussed. In addition, the text is enriched by numerous real-life quotes from tutors, students and employers. This is, without doubt, an extremely useful addition to the series that future nursing students, college tutors and careers advisers will find invaluable.

Professor Shirley Bach
Series Editor
December 2014

Acknowledgements

The author and publishers would like to thank the Department of Health for permission to reproduce material from *Nursing Careers Framework Poster* (Department of Health 2010) in Table 1.2.

From the authors:

Thank you to the students, mentors, practice colleagues and our service users and role players for their contributions to the book. Martyn Keen thanks Lucy Riddett and Stefanie Looker in particular.

Jon – for all your support and endless cups of tea and coffee.

Introduction

Who is this book for?

If you are interested in becoming a nurse or your work involves helping people to choose a career or apply to university then this book has been written for you. While primarily aimed at those actually considering a career in nursing, the information in here will be of interest to careers advisers, parents, schools and colleges. This book will guide you through the key steps of applying to university, from making the initial decision as to whether nursing is the right career choice for you and whether you are right for nursing through to the application process, entry tests and selection days, finishing with how to prepare in the months leading up to the start of the programme. It will provide you with down-to-earth, practical help and advice that will help you to increase your chance of success.

Why *Getting into Nursing*?

Nursing is one of the most popular courses applied for at universities, receiving the highest number of applications (226,400) of all university courses in 2013 with over nine applications for every place offered. While the number of places universities offer for nursing programmes varies each year depending on the need for nurses within the NHS, the general trend over the last few years is a year on year increase in the numbers of candidates applying. Since 2013 nursing has become an all degree profession offering only BSc(Hons) and postgraduate programmes.

Following a series of healthcare scandals in recent years universities have been required to make significant changes to their recruitment and selection processes and are now using values-based recruitment methods to ensure the right people with the right values and behaviours are recruited. The whole selection and interview process is now therefore more challenging than in the past. In light of all these factors it is likely that the competition for a place on a nursing course will not only increase, but also mean that applicants will need to be far better prepared in order to be successful. The aim of this book is to help you achieve your aim of 'getting into nursing'.

Book structure

Chapter 1 aims to clarify the nurse's role and correct the many misconceptions held about nursing by the public and the media. It will introduce you to the four fields of nursing (adult, children's, learning disabilities and mental health), look at the different environments in which nurses work and has updated the possible career pathways open to you once you have successfully completed your course to reflect recent changes in the way healthcare is being delivered.

Chapter 2 examines what is required and expected of a nurse in terms of personal attributes, values and skills from a range of different perspectives, including the professional body that sets the standards for nurses and nursing, the patients who are recipients of nursing care, the expectations of the Chief Nurse for England and the people who employ nurses at the end of their programme. It challenges you to consider whether you have the right qualities to become a nurse. It also sets out to allay the fear that people with a disability may have that nursing could never be a career for them and explains the implications of having a criminal record if you wish to become a nurse.

Chapter 3 describes the specific academic entry requirements for nursing programmes and looks at the other attributes you will need to demonstrate to enhance your application. For those without standard academic qualifications, alternative routes into nursing are explored.

Chapter 4 looks at the different types of work experience and voluntary work that you may wish to consider undertaking prior to applying for nursing in order to improve your chances of being successful in your application and at interview. This chapter also looks at how you can demonstrate how the job you are currently doing can demonstrate that you have the right values and behaviours that universities are looking for.

Chapter 5 explores what is involved in studying for a nursing qualification and how a nursing degree or postgraduate course differs from more traditional subjects that can be studied at university. You will get an insight into how a nursing programme is structured to enable you to gain both the theoretical knowledge and the practical experience you will require in order to meet the requirements of the course. The practicalities of undertaking a nursing course are explored, such as attendance, the importance of professional behaviour and placement learning opportunities.

Chapter 6 looks at the four fields of nursing: adult, child health, mental health and learning disability nursing. The aim is to help you appreciate the differences between them by describing how the type of work nurses undertake in each field differs and the different environments, so that you can strengthen your personal statement for your chosen field. Suggestions are also given for the different types of voluntary or work experiences that you can choose to help support your application for your chosen field.

Chapter 7 describes the process for applying for a nursing course at university through UCAS. The first decision to be made is which universities to put on your application form and so this chapter looks at the information available to you, such as league tables, student websites and the national student survey, which can help inform your choice. Practical considerations such as travel, money and the availability of disability support are also looked at, as these can be barriers to success once you are on the course if not considered in advance.

Chapter 8 helps you to prepare for your nursing selection day on a practical level. Questions such as 'What preparation do I need to undertake?', 'What do I need to take with me?' and 'What should I wear?' are all addressed.

Chapter 9 tackles the thorny problem of numeracy tests, which many universities now use as part of their selection process. This chapter looks at the different types of calculations you are likely to see in numeracy tests and explains why numeracy is an important skill for nurses to have. Example test papers are offered to enable you to practise your skills.

Chapter 10 looks at why literacy skills are important in nursing and why universities test for it on selection days. It aims to deepen your understanding of the specific skills required so that you can appreciate what is expected of you when applying to university, during your course and later when applying for your first post and provides examples of the many different literacy tests used by universities.

Chapter 11 focuses on the selection day. It explores the many different ways that applicants are selected for a nursing degree programme, from interviews to group discussions and role play and the increased focus on values-based recruitment. An insight into the qualities that universities are looking for is given and some of the common mistakes made by candidates at selection days are looked at, with guidance given on how to avoid them.

The last chapter describes what happens after you have been offered a place or what to do if you are unsuccessful. It takes you through the next steps both by UCAS and the university and what you can do to put yourself in the best position for your studies before you start as well as the practicalities of finding accommodation. If you don't get an offer the options open to you are explored, from reapplying to other universities to gaining additional qualifications or work experience.

Throughout the book, you will find the terms 'patient', 'service user' and 'client' used according to the field of nursing and setting being described. Most people who use mental health and learning disability services prefer to be called service users rather than patients.

Learning features and activities

You can read this book from cover to cover or you may just wish to dip into certain chapters depending where you are in the process of applying for a nursing course. Throughout the book you will find activities that will help you to prepare for the application and selection process as well as considering the practicalities about which university is right for you.

All the activities require you to take a break from reading the text: some just require you to reflect on your own skills and abilities, while others require access to the internet. There are also top tips provided by students and lecturers to help you both before and after starting your course as well as recommended reading and websites that can provide more information if you want to explore a particular area in more detail. Many of these activities will prepare you for writing your personal statement, which is key to getting selected for an interview, as well as helping to prepare you for your selection day.

The Appendix provides you with a visual timeline of the whole process of applying to university and refers back to the relevant chapters for each stage to help you keep on track.

Chapter 1
What is nursing today?

Karen Elcock

Chapter aims

The aim of this chapter is to clarify the role of the nurse and how different people view nursing. By the end of this chapter you will be able to:

- describe the role of the nurse;
- describe the different fields of practice in which nurses work;
- appreciate the wide variety of places where nursing takes place;
- demonstrate insight into the varied career pathways nurses can follow.

Introduction

One of the most popular questions most likely to be posed at interview for a place on a nursing course is: 'What do you think the role of the nurse is?' While you would expect someone applying for a nursing programme to have a very clear idea of what a nurse is and what nurses do, it is surprising how many applicants struggle to answer this question well. Common answers tend to be along the lines of 'caring for patients', 'giving drugs' and 'helping patients get better'. While each of these is true, nursing is so much more than this. This chapter explores the role of the nurse and helps you to gain a clearer picture of what nurses do and the many career opportunities open to you once you qualify.

Activity 1.1   *What is the role of the nurse?*

NHS Careers has a range of videos about nursing which give you some interesting insights. A good one to start with is *Myth busting* (**http://nursing.nhscareers.nhs.uk/why/myth_busting**).

- How many of these misconceptions did you hold?
- Has your view of nursing changed at all?

If you cannot access the internet, jot down what you think the role of the nurse is.

What is nursing?

You would think this would be an easy question to answer but, believe it or not, even nurses themselves struggle to describe exactly what their role is, partly because the role is so varied, but also because so much of their role is hidden and difficult to quantify.

Christine Beasley, when Chief Nursing Officer for England, identified the problem well when she said:

> *Nursing may not always be easy to describe but patients know when they get good nursing, and when they do not. Nursing requires a high level set of skills and understanding which, taken separately, may seem commonplace and undemanding, but combined as a whole is far more complex and powerful.*
> (Department of Health, 2006, p4)

If you ask the public you will find there are many different views, and it is likely that when you have told people that you are applying for nursing you will have received responses that reflect these views. Bridges (1990) described four stereotypes:

1. the ministering angel;
2. the battleaxe;
3. the naughty nurse;
4. the doctor's handmaiden.

Many of these views of nurses have been influenced by the media. For example, the *Carry On* films and the book and film *One Flew Over the Cuckoo's Nest* portray nurses as bossy, matriarchal types. Television programmes such as *No Angels* promote the naughty nurse image and this is further promoted in the tabloid press and with the availability of fancy dress nursing uniforms, which are invariably skimpy. Television series such as *House, Grey's Anatomy* and *ER* perpetuate the myth that nurses are just there to serve doctors – a myth some doctors still believe. The nurse as ministering angel, typified by the image of Florence Nightingale and the lamp, is also a popular one, also promoted in the press, although regular reports of poor care have changed the views of some.

The definition of nursing most commonly cited was written by Virginia Henderson in the 1960s, but is still as relevant today.

Definition of nursing

> *[T]o assist the individual, sick or well, in the performance of those activities contributing to health or its recovery (or to peaceful death) that he would perform unaided if he had the necessary strength, will, or knowledge. And to do this in such a way as to help him gain independence as rapidly as possible. This aspect of her work, this part of her function, she initiates and controls; of this she is master. In addition she helps the patient to carry out the therapeutic plan as initiated by the physician. She also, as a member of a team, helps others as they in turn help her, to plan and carry out the total program whether it be for the improvement of health, or recovery from illness, or support in death.*
> (Henderson, 1966, p15)

Henderson's definition is important as not only does it highlight that nursing isn't just about helping people to get better, but also it describes the nurse as someone who works with the patient (rather than just 'doing to'), is a team player and certainly isn't just someone who does what he or she is told. This was a fairly advanced view in the 1960s.

The Nursing and Midwifery Council (NMC) and your nursing career

It is important for your future career in nursing, and to prepare for your selection day, that you appreciate the role of the NMC. The NMC is the nursing and midwifery regulator for England, Wales, Scotland, Northern Ireland and the islands. Its role is:

- to safeguard the health and wellbeing of the public;
- to set standards of education, training, conduct and performance so that nurses and midwives can deliver high-quality healthcare consistently throughout their careers;
- to ensure that nurses and midwives keep their skills and knowledge up to date and uphold professional standards;
- to have clear and transparent processes to investigate nurses and midwives who fall short of NMC standards (**www.nmc-uk.org**).

If you are successful, at the end of your pre-registration nursing programme you will be eligible to be added to the register of nurses and midwives held by the NMC and can then call yourself a 'registered nurse'. Each registered nurse has a unique personal identification number, or PIN, and this is required for you to work as a nurse or midwife in the UK. Registered nurses renew their registration every three years and are required to have kept their knowledge and skills up to date. In order to renew their registration, registered nurses have to assure the NMC that they have worked as a nurse for a required number of hours over the previous three years and undertaken a specified amount of study relevant to their practice. The aim is to ensure that all practising nurses keep up to date in both theory and practice. So becoming a nurse is not just about getting the degree – it is a commitment to lifetime learning.

The registered nurse qualification is recognised in the UK and throughout the European Union and has a good reputation overseas. Many nurses will tell you that it is a huge privilege and honour to become a nurse and that there is a range of career opportunities available to you once you have become a registered nurse, in the UK and abroad, and in the NHS, private and voluntary sectors of healthcare. The world is your oyster!

All registered nurses must all work in line with *The Code* (Nursing and Midwifery Council, 2015). This code lays down the standards of conduct, performance and ethics for nurses and midwives. A word of caution, here: as well as being added to the register, nurses can also be removed from it if their 'fitness to practise' as a nurse is questioned and then proved to be unacceptable. You will find that we will keep coming back to the importance of professionalism throughout this book because entering nursing is not like entering most other jobs: people's lives will depend on you and if you are to engender their trust then the way you behave both at work and in your personal life has to be in a way that fosters that trust.

The fields of nursing

You may be wondering what a 'field' has to do with nursing, or why there should be lots of fields with nurses in them. The NMC, which sets the standards for nursing education programmes, uses the term to describe the four main areas in which nurses specialise:

- adult nursing: the care of people aged 18 or over;
- children's nursing: the care of children and young people from birth to late teens;
- learning disabilities nursing: the care of people of all ages who have learning disabilities;
- mental health nursing: the care of people of all ages who have mental health problems (**www.nmc-uk.org**).

If you want to undertake a pre-registration nursing course you will need to decide which field of practice you wish to specialise in before you even start the application process, as you will be applying to follow a programme that leads to registration as a nurse in one of those fields. Some universities offer joint qualifications, enabling you to register in two fields of practice at the end of the programme, e.g. registered nurse (adult) and registered nurse (child), but these programmes are longer to enable you to gain the practice experience and theory input to meet the learning outcomes for both fields of practice.

Chapter 6 has more detailed information about the different fields and is worth reading before you make your final decision.

Where does nursing take place?

Traditionally nursing has been seen as taking place primarily in hospitals, but nursing in fact takes place wherever people live, work, play or are educated (**www.nmc-uk.org**). Table 1.1 lists some of the places where nurses deliver care. It is crudely divided between hospital/inpatient-based settings and community settings, but in reality many nurses work across the inpatient–community boundary. It should also be noted that many of these settings are as likely to be part of a private or independent organisation as they are to be part of the NHS. The NHS has seen significant changes in the demographics of the people who require its services in recent years. People are living longer so there is not only an increase in the number of older people requiring care, but also a concurrent increase in the number of people with dementia and long-term conditions. As a consequence more care will be delivered in the community and in people's homes in the future and many newly qualified nurses are therefore going into the community for their first posts.

Careers in nursing

Nursing as a career choice endows these professionals with a range of skills that can enhance all facets of their life. Nurses with compassion and humanity bring these attributes into many other areas such as family, friends and social life. The enhanced communication skills required make nurses at ease in any social situation and able to converse with people from all backgrounds and walks of life. The skills and knowledge gained in their working life are entirely portable, allowing nurses to practise in very different settings and with many different patient groups. Career choices, such as research, education or management along with clinical practice, allow career progression and specialist interests rarely afforded in other professions. The diversity of practice environments are vast and provide an interesting, rewarding and stimulating career that lasts a lifetime.

(Elizabeth Robb, Chief Executive, The Florence Nightingale Foundation)

Adult	Child	Learning disability	Mental health
Hospital/inpatient-based			
Medical/surgical units/wards	Medical/surgical wards	Treatment and wards	Inpatient assessment units
Operating departments	Operating departments	Forensic services	Rehabilitation wards
Outpatients departments	Outpatients departments	Dual disability inpatient services	Forensic units
Accident and emergency departments	Accident and emergency departments	Prisons	Accident and emergency departments
Critical care units	Critical care units		Intensive care units
Prisons	Day care units		Prisons
Day care units			
Community-based			
At home	At home	At home	At home
GP/health centres	GP/health centres	Community learning disability teams	Community mental health teams
Schools	Schools	Schools	Day units
Urgent care/walk-in centres	Urgent care/walk-in centres	Special schools	Substance misuse services

(Continued)

(Continued)

NHS 111/NHS 24 NHS direct Wales	NHS 111/NHS 24 NHS direct Wales	Supported living schemes	Nursing homes
Occupational health departments	Child and maternal health services	Child and maternal health services	Child and maternal health services
Nursing homes	Hospice	GP practices	GP practices
Hospice		Residential homes	Therapeutic day services
		Day services	

Table 1.1: Where nursing takes place

Once qualified, nursing offers a wide range of career pathways. While you do not have to decide before you start your course where you want your career to go, you may be asked at interview where you see yourself in five years' time or how you see your career progressing, so having some idea will help you to answer those questions if they arise. In reality, many students change their minds as they progress through their course and have different practice experiences.

Activity 1.2   *Nursing careers*

The Department of Health has developed a visual framework to help nurses plan their careers and NHS employers have built an interactive website around the framework to help you explore possible career options. Visit the website: **http://nursingcareers.nhsemployers. org** and browse the framework.

- Has it changed your views about possible careers in nursing?
- What would your answer now be if asked where you saw your career in five years' time?

Make a note of it in preparation for your interview.

Table 1.2 offers a simplified version of the careers framework. The framework provides an insight into a very small number of possible career pathways available to you once you qualify.

Many nurses will move between pathways of care, for example working in an acute ward and then moving into a role in the community supporting people with long-term conditions. They may also move between the role dimensions, for example from a clinical role to a management role to an education or research role over their career lifetime. The case study on page 14 gives an example of this.

Pathways of care	Role dimensions			
	Clinical	Research	Management	Education
First contact, access and urgent care	Staff nurse	Clinical research staff nurse	Project leader	Practice education facilitator
	Senior staff nurse Practice nurse Nurse telephone adviser	Research assistant	Team leader Project manager	Lecturer practitioner
	Nurse practitioner Senior nurse walk-in/urgent care centre	Clinical trials nurse Research fellow	Service manager	Senior lecturer
	Named nurse child protection	Reader	Service development and governance manager	Head of department
	Practice partner	Professor	Board director Chief executive officer	University dean
Acute and critical care	Staff nurse	Clinical research staff nurse	Project leader	Practice education facilitator
	Senior staff nurse Nurse practitioner	Research assistant	Team leader	Lecturer practitioner
	Nurse practitioner Surgical care practitioner	Clinical trials nurse Research fellow	Ward sister/charge nurse Service manager	Senior lecturer
	Paediatric advanced nurse practitioner Nurse consultant	Reader	Theatre manager Modern matron	Head of department
	Clinical professor	Professor	Policy adviser Board director	University dean

(Continued)

(Continued)

Pathways of care	Role dimensions			
	Clinical	Research	Management	Education
Family and public health	Community staff nurse	Clinical research staff nurse	Project manager	Practice education facilitator
	Occupational health nurse Community staff nurse Practice nurse	Research assistant	Project manager	Lecturer practitioner
	Health visitor School nurse Family partnership nurse	Clinical trials nurse Research fellow	Community team leader Service manager	Senior lecturer
	Consultant health visitor	Reader	Lead practice nurse Assistant director community services	Head of department
	Director of public health	Professor	Policy adviser	University dean
Mental health and psycho-social care	Staff nurse	Clinical research staff nurse	Project manager	Practice education facilitator
	Community mental health nurse Community learning disabilities nurse	Research assistant	Team leader	Lecturer practitioner
	Clinical nurse specialist Community mental health nurse	Clinical trials nurse Research fellow	Ward manager Nurse adviser	Senior lecturer

Table 1.2: Nursing career pathways

	Nurse consultant	Reader	Lead nurse (learning disabilities) Assistant director (mental health)	Head of department
	Clinical professor mental health	Professor	Board director	University dean
Supporting long-term care	Community staff nurse Residential care home nurse	Clinical research staff nurse	Project manager – long-term conditions	Clinical education facilitator
	District nurse Practice nurse	Research assistant	Team leader – long-term conditions	Lecturer practitioner
	Clinical nurse specialist	Clinical trials nurse Research fellow	Community team manager Service manager – long-term care	Senior lecturer
	Nurse consultant	Reader	Community matron	Head of department
	Practice partner	Professor	Board director	University dean

Table 1.2: Nursing career pathways

Source: adapted from Department of Health, 2010.

Case study

Professor Vari Drennan, registered nurse and registered specialist community public health practitioner, Associate Dean for Research; Professor of Health Policy and Service Delivery says:

I work as Professor of Health Policy and my passion is to understand how we can improve healthcare and social care in the community. My job is to provide that information and ideas to people who can make that difference.

I came to nursing from a Saturday job as a care assistant, caring for frail and disabled older people in a nursing home. I undertook an innovative course that focused me on public health and community health, qualifying as a registered nurse, a registered health visitor and with a degree in sociology and social administration. My first post as a staff nurse on a medical ward in Southampton University led me to understand why attention to preventive public health was so important at an individual and family level. My second post was as a health visitor in the vibrant, ethnically diverse and, at that time, very deprived area around Portobello Road, London. My daily working life demonstrated the levels of inequalities in people's lives and health experiences and that by critically examining how we practised and provided healthcare we could make changes at some levels. I took every opportunity offered to enquire into how we could better provide our services, working as a research health visitor on projects aimed at preventive healthcare for older people and using community development techniques (and gained my Master's degree).

I moved into a teaching post (and gained a teaching qualification) to share my knowledge, also publishing a book called Health Visiting and Groups: Politics and practice, *as a way of sharing information with my wider peers. I returned to the health service as a professional development nurse in Islington, London, community health service, i.e. someone employed to support other nurses and staff to improve practice and services. I took every opportunity offered to me and I became more involved in the management of the services. I went on to become both a senior community health service manager and a head of community nursing (gaining management qualifications). I was leading on innovative ways to improve the quality of our services and working as part of a team in responding to new forms of contracting and growing financial pressures.*

I moved to a university post (University College London) when an opportunity arose to lead on research into how best to provide nursing and health visiting in primary care. At the same time I also undertook front-line clinical practice again. I completed my PhD and co-wrote books for primary care professionals on primary care for older people and primary care and dementia with a general practitioner. My research into community nursing workforce was commissioned and used by the Department of Health (England). In my post in Kingston University and St George's, University of London, I am undertaking government-funded research into a range of primary care issues; I teach as well as support nurses and others to learn how to undertake research. My job is to support and nurture 'enquiring minds', which I think are the bedrock for improving the types and quality of health and nursing services.

Nursing has given me the opportunity for a rich and varied career – it offers many opportunities and routes for people with all types of interests and passions.

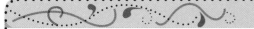

Chapter summary

Out of all the career options available to you, nursing possibly provides the greatest range of opportunities. Once qualified, you can work in a large hospital, in the community, in teams or alone, remain clinically focused or move into management, research or education, stay in the UK or work abroad. It is not, however, a career for everyone and the next chapter will help you determine whether you have the skills and attributes required to join what is one of the most rewarding jobs available.

Further reading

Commissioning Board Chief Nursing Officer and DH Chief Nursing Adviser (2012) *Compassion in Practice: Nursing, midwifery and care staff – our vision and strategy.* Available from: **www.england.nhs. uk/wp-content/uploads/2012/12/compassion-in-practice.pdf**

This is the vision and strategy for nursing and midwifery published in 2012 to ensure delivery of high quality compassionate care. Includes information on the 6Cs.

Hall, C and Ritchie, D (2013) *What is Nursing? Exploring theory and practice,* 3rd edition. London: Sage/ Learning Matters.

A really useful overview of nursing, both nationally and internationally, and includes excellent first-hand accounts of what it is like to be a registered nurse in the different fields of nursing.

Useful websites

http://nursing.nhscareers.nhs.uk

NHS nursing careers website that contains really useful information about nursing with excellent videos and other resources.

http://nursingcareers.nhsemployers.org

Career Planner for Nurses is a website that provides an interactive tool to explore different career pathways in nursing and provides a number of case studies of different roles at all levels and fields of practice.

www.nmc-uk.org

Nursing and Midwifery Council website.

Chapter 2
Do I have what it takes to be a nurse?

Karen Elcock

Chapter aims

The aim of this chapter is to explore whether you have got what it takes to become a nurse. By the end of this chapter you will be able to:

- understand what is expected of a nurse by the Nursing and Midwifery Council (NMC), patients and employers;
- list the personal attributes, values and skills required of a nurse and consider whether you have them;
- appreciate the challenges that undertaking a nursing degree may pose for you;
- understand how universities and healthcare settings support students with a disability.

Introduction

A good nurse is one who understands that compassion and caring are vital attributes in a first-class nurse. It is a privilege to care for people at some of the most vulnerable times in their lives and to do so requires a high level of skill, knowledge and expertise which nurse training brings. All of this is combined to make a worthwhile and interesting career choice for those who truly wish to combine undergraduate scientific education with excellent communication skills in a caring profession.
(Elizabeth Robb, Chief Executive, The Florence Nightingale Foundation)

Chapter 1 focused on what nursing is and what nurses do. If you are reading this chapter then you are still interested, but may be wondering whether you have 'got what it takes' to be a nurse. If you've discussed your interest in nursing with others it is quite likely that at least one person has said: 'I could never do a job like that'. It is certainly true that nursing is not something that will suit everyone, but it is also true that not everyone is suitable to do nursing. This chapter will help you decide whether you have got what it takes to be a nurse.

What attributes, values and skills does a nurse need?

There is a general perception that the main qualities you need to become a nurse are to be kind and caring, and it has often been seen as a good job for people who were less academic at school.

Nurses certainly need to demonstrate kindness and caring, and students enter nursing with a range of academic abilities, which we will discuss in the next chapter. However, a lot more is required from nurses today than in the past and you will need to be able to demonstrate that you have the range of personal attributes, values and skills that are required as well as the ability to undertake what will be a challenging, but ultimately rewarding, course. You may have heard about the healthcare scandals at Mid Staffordshire Hospital which were reported in the media and which led to a public inquiry by Robert Francis QC. One of the recommendations in his report (Francis, 2013) was the need to ensure that universities select people who wish to become nurses who have the right values and behaviours. We will come back to this again in this chapter and later chapters as the report has led to significant changes in the way that universities now select student nurses.

You have probably considered why you wish to become a nurse, but have you considered what you have to offer nursing? Activity 2.1 will start you off.

Activity 2.1 **Your personal attributes, values and skills**

In considering nursing as a career you must have thought about what you have to offer.

List the personal attributes, values and skills that you believe you have that would make you a good nurse. Consider feedback you have had from school/college, friends, family and employers.

Keep this list and we will return to it later.

You will have ideas about what makes a good nurse, but in order to sell yourself on your application form and at interview you will need to be able to convince the university that you appreciate which attributes are important and are able to demonstrate that you have them. Universities will have their own views about what attributes are essential and these will have been developed in consultation with patients, service users (the term commonly used for people who use mental health or learning disability services) and carers, and the healthcare organisations with which the universities work and which may offer you employment at the end of your programme. In addition, the NMC has very clear requirements with regard to the skills, knowledge and values that are required of a nurse. We will therefore look at what is expected of a nurse from a number of different perspectives to give you a feel of what will be expected of you.

The NMC's perspective

The NMC is the organisation with which all nurses must register in order to practise as a registered nurse in the UK and have several roles (see box on page 18).

Nursing and Midwifery Council

The role of the NMC is:

- to safeguard the health and well-being of the public;
- to set standards of education, training, conduct and performance so that nurses and midwives can deliver high-quality healthcare consistently throughout their career;
- to ensure that nurses and midwives keep their skills and knowledge up to date and uphold professional standards;
- to have clear and transparent processes to investigate nurses and midwives who fall short of NMC standards (**www.nmc-uk.org**).

The NMC set the Standards for Pre-registration Nursing Education (Nursing and Midwifery Council, 2010), against which universities develop their pre-registration nursing programmes. These are quite lengthy but set out standards of competence, which describe the knowledge, skills and attitudes that nurses must attain by the end of the programme before they are allowed to register as a nurse. However, whilst the focus of the standards is on what you must acquire and demonstrate by the end of the programme, you will need to be able to demonstrate that you already possess some of the expected knowledge, skills and attitudes in your application form and at interview.

The key skills and attributes within the NMC's standards include:

- compassion;
- respect for others;
- integrity;
- caring;
- being non-judgmental;
- sensitivity to others;
- ability to identify own limitations;
- excellent communication and interpersonal skills;
- empathy;
- adaptability;
- flexibility;
- team worker.

A graduate registered nurse is a safe, caring, and competent decision maker willing to accept personal and professional accountability for his/her actions and continuous learning. The nurse practises within a statutory framework and code of ethics delivering nursing practice (care) that is

appropriately based on research, evidence and critical thinking that effectively responds to the needs of individual clients (patients) and diverse populations.
(Nursing and Midwifery Council, 2010)

In addition the NMC places particular emphasis on good character, specifically that you should be honest and trustworthy. The NMC provides guidance for nurses on their conduct in *The Code: Professional standards of practice and behaviour for nurses and midwives* (Nursing and Midwifery Council, 2015), which is worth reading as it sets out expectations of the nurse and the professional code which you would be expected to follow both as a student nurse and in your personal life. Again a key focus in this guidance is the importance of a student nurse being both honest and trustworthy. How you behave in your personal life may be something that you had not considered as being either important or relevant to a job you may hold. However in nursing your behaviour in your personal life can have direct consequences for your continuation on a nursing programme or for your job once you register as a nurse. At all times you will be representing the nursing profession and therefore your conduct must never bring the profession into disrepute. There is further information about this on the NMC website (**www.nmc-uk.org**) and we will look at the importance of good character in more depth in Chapter 3.

The perspective of patients and service users

Universities work very closely with patients, service users and carers to ensure that their programmes will develop nurses that meet their expectations. In some universities, patients and service users are also involved in their selection days (see Chapter 11). Nurses play a significant role in the care of patients and service users, particularly in the hospital environment where nurses are the only healthcare professionals in contact with them 24 hours a day. Increasingly, however, nurses are the first point of contact in the community, walk-in centres and at GP surgeries and so are delivering a far wider service to patients and service users than in the past.

The expectations of patients and service users will vary, dependent on the point they come into contact with you and their particular needs at that time. However some basic expectations have been identified:

- to be treated as an individual;
- to be involved in their care;
- nurses care for and care about them;
- compassionate care;
- nurses possess effective communication skills (Maben and Griffiths, 2008).

The extracts below provide personal views of patients and service users about what they expect of a nurse. They cover each of the four fields of practice in nursing.

The employers' perspective

Unfortunately it is not a foregone conclusion that a job will be waiting for you at the end of your programme. You will probably be competing for a post against colleagues from your own university as well as from other universities. Many organisations now require candidates not only to attend an interview, but also to sit numeracy and literacy tests and even participate in skills assessments. In a competitive market it will therefore be imperative that you have demonstrated your commitment to nursing whilst undertaking your degree and can demonstrate that you have the skills required. In a study undertaken in 2010 (Ooms, 2011), the key attributes expected of a nurse by NHS trusts in London were:

- good communication skills;
- teamwork skills;
- common sense;
- flexibility;
- awareness of own limitations;
- enthusiasm to learn;
- ability to prioritise;
- professional attitude;
- good clinical judgment;
- good core clinical skills;
- awareness of equality and diversity issues.

While the last four are skills that you will develop by undertaking your nursing programme, the first seven are ones that you should already possess to a greater or lesser degree and will be able to develop further during your programme.

As a Trust we want to employ newly qualified nurses who are knowledgeable doers. In that we mean a nurse who is competent to deliver safe care to patients in a kind, considerate and empathetic

manner that acknowledges individual needs. In a nutshell as a Trust we need nurses who possess the ingredients listed on the label to be able to deliver patient-centred care. There is no point in opening up a tin of tomatoes to find the content is condensed milk when you wanted the tomatoes to make spaghetti bolognaise.
(Sarah, Professional Development Lead, Acute Trust)

The university's perspective

The university you apply to will have expectations of you based not only on those that have been discussed from the different stakeholder perspectives above, but also in relation to your commitment to the programme. At interview you will be expected to demonstrate not only that you have the required knowledge, skills and attributes to be a nurse, but also that you understand what nursing is and have considered what it means in terms of commitment for you and your ability to meet those commitments. Each university has a different interview process and we will explore this in more depth in Chapter 11, but key areas about you, as a person, that they will be looking for are:

- effective communication skills;

- good time management skills;

- insight and self-awareness of strengths and weaknesses;

- team-working skills;

- how you manage stress/difficult situations;

- an understanding of skills you will need to learn both in the university and out in practice.

Lecturer view . . . I look for someone who can communicate well, has done their homework and understands what nursing is about (the downsides as well as the ups) and can demonstrate that they have the resilience to undertake what is a tough course compared to many other degrees.

As you will have seen by now, the different stakeholders have common expectations, in particular:

- excellent communication and interpersonal skills;

- team worker;

- compassion and caring;

- respect for others/treating people as individuals;

- insight and self-awareness of strengths and weaknesses.

However, in response to the Francis Report mentioned earlier, Jane Cummings, the Chief Nursing Officer for England along with Viv Bennett, Director of Nursing at the Department of

Health, developed a vision for nursing underpinned by what are known as the 6Cs. Some of these are identified above (care, compassion and communication) but there are three more and you will therefore find that universities will be looking for candidates who can demonstrate all of these values and behaviours through their personal statement and at interview.

Activity 2.2 will help you to review whether you have these skills, attributes and values.

Activity 2.2

Do I have the required skills, attributes and values to be a nurse?

The skills, attributes and values that seem to be common to the different groups above along with the 6Cs are listed in the table below. Compare them to the ones you identified in Activity 2.1. Which ones do you already possess?

	Yes	No	Maybe
Team worker	✓		
Respect for others/treating people as individuals	✓		
Insight and self-awareness of strengths and weaknesses	✓		
Care	✓		
Compassion	✓		
Competence	✓		
Communication	✓		
Courage	✓		
Commitment	✓		

If you already have many of the attributes, skills and values expected of a nurse, well done; you are off to a good start. If you are unsure then talk to others and get their honest opinion. What will be important is how you provide evidence of each of these or discuss how the course will help you develop them. We will look at preparing your personal statement in Chapter 7 and how you can provide evidence of the areas you have identified in this chapter.

The challenges of a nursing programme

As well as having the academic qualifications and the attributes, skills and values discussed above, you will need to appreciate how challenging undertaking a nursing degree programme will be.

It is important that you have thought through whether you can manage the challenges you will face, which will not only be academic ones but also personal ones. Being a nursing student is very different from being a traditional university student who spends up to 15 hours a week at university between October and June. The challenge of a nursing programme is that not only do you have to meet the academic requirements of a degree programme, but on top of that you will be required to undertake a minimum of 2300 hours of practice learning experiences over the course of the programme. As a consequence your course is really packed and you will have less free time and fewer holidays and will need to be able to manage your time well to meet the course requirements, both academic and out in practice.

So you need to consider whether you can manage the following:

- attend practice for 37.5 hours a week (on average);
- travel to different practice learning areas, sometimes across a wide geographical area;
- undertake a range of different shifts (this is an NMC requirement), e.g.:
  - shifts that start as early as 7.30 a.m.;
  - shifts that end late in the evening;
  - weekend shifts;
  - night duty;
- cope with the physical and emotional demands when out in practice;
- accept that in some fields of nursing the majority of your patients/service users will be elderly and many will have dementia;
- care for people who are distressed, frightened, angry or demanding;
- deal with difficult moral and ethical issues that may not result in outcomes you feel are right;
- continue to study after a hard day in practice;
- have limited time off in the school holidays;
- be able to meet deadlines for assessments (these could number six or more per year).

It is important to remember that, while the above are some of the challenges you will face, they will be balanced by the enjoyment you get from learning about nursing and being involved in the care of patients and service users. The comment from students below about their experiences on a pre-registration nursing programme shows this balance.

Students' views . . . Nursing is just the best but it is incredibly hard work as you have to study even while you are on practice placements and the different shifts play havoc with your personal and social life. However, all of this is forgotten when you pass an assignment or when you have had a really hard day and a patient turns round and says 'thank you for

continued . . .

listening to me'. You know you've made a difference to someone's life and not many people get a chance to do that (third-year student).

If nursing is what you really, really want to do, then go for it. But, before you invest three years of your life studying to become one, be absolutely sure it's for you. Be aware that it makes huge demands on stamina and that you have to take the rough with the smooth. Nothing good comes easy; be prepared for real challenges and brace yourself for it (Gavin, David and Christiana – student nurses).

Mature students

Nursing attracts a large number of mature students (the average age is over 25 years, with many students in their 30s–50s and older). The challenges for many mature students are around juggling family commitments. Managing family commitments means you will need good support mechanisms, particularly around childcare both on a day-to-day basis and during school holidays. Remember you will be leaving home very early in the morning and often not getting home until very late at night, plus working at weekends and in the school holidays, so consider how you will manage this.

The good news is that thousands of mature students qualify every year, but you will need to be organised, plan ahead and be willing to call on help and support from family and friends to help you through your studies.

Student tip . . . When I was looking into nursing programmes I found that there were a number of student nurse forums and blogs on the internet that gave me some really useful insights into the challenges and joys of nursing (e.g. the Student Room). Some of the forums had people asking questions about nursing as a career, others asked each other about different universities and their interview processes. Obviously you need to take into consideration that people may not always be honest, but there can be some useful nuggets of information available and I'd strongly recommend taking a look at them.

Finances

One of the causes often given by students for deciding to leave a nursing programme is financial. Although your university fees are currently paid and there is some financial support through grants and bursaries, it can still be difficult to manage. Many students do additional paid work, but it has to be flexible to fit round your programme and your time in clinical practice. It is also important that it does not have an impact on your ability to study and meet course requirements. Each country in the UK has its own bursary unit and their websites are given at the end of the chapter. The types of help that may be available to you are:

- payment of course fees;
- non-means-tested grant;
- means-tested bursary;
- maintenance loan;
- initial expenses allowance;
- dependants' allowance;
- single parents' allowance;
- childcare allowance for parents;
- disabled students' allowance;
- expenses for travelling to clinical placements.

Note that these may vary slightly for each country and are constantly under review and liable to change, so you are strongly recommended to look at what financial help you might receive and consider how you would survive on this amount. Take into consideration your fares to and from university and out to your practice placements. You can currently be reimbursed the additional cost for travel to placements if it costs more than travelling to university, but you will need to pay these costs first and then be reimbursed. Activity 2.3 will help you assess whether you can afford the travel costs and times for your nursing course.

Activity 2.3	*Travel costs*

Look at the websites of the main universities you are interested in. Find out where they are based and which hospitals and trusts they work in partnership with. Use the internet to find out how long it will take to travel to different sites by car or use travel timetables for public transport. Work out what time you would need to leave home (or university/local accommodation) to get to the different hospitals/trusts by 7.15 a.m., 1 p.m. and 9 p.m. Then find out what time you would get back home if you leave your placement at 7.30 a.m., 4 p.m. and 9 p.m. Do this for weekdays, Saturdays and Sundays. Then work out the costs based on five week-day shifts.

Questions to ask yourself are: Can I manage the travel times? Can I afford the fares/petrol? Can I get to placements on a Sunday?

Student tip … I would genuinely advise new students who have been in employment to go part-time for at least two months after starting university before finally resigning. This is to avoid undue financial pressure at the start of the programme (Christine).

Getting an insight into nursing

In order to be sure that nursing is the right career path, you will find it very useful to gain some experience in a relevant health or social care setting before studying. In this way you will gain an insight into healthcare and meet other qualified healthcare professionals, which gives you the opportunity to see what their work involves and talk to them about their experiences. We explore more about how you can gain work experience in Chapter 4.

Is nursing possible if I have a health condition or a disability?

The NMC requires all nurses to have good health in order to provide safe and effective practice. This does not mean that if you have a health condition or a disability you cannot become a nurse. All applicants to a nursing programme who declare a health condition or disability will be assessed where appropriate by an occupational health department and/or be referred to the disability support team at the university. The disability team can then explore with you what reasonable adjustments you might need to enable you to undertake the programme both within the university and out in practice. All universities will have a disability support team and you should find that they will take enquiries from prospective students, which means you can contact them in advance with any questions and these will be treated in full confidence.

The Equality Act (2010) aims to protect people with a disability as well as prevent discrimination. It includes legal rights for people with a disability, including those who are in education (Office for Disability Issues, 2011). Under the Act a person has *a disability if he or she has a physical or mental impairment and the impairment has a substantial and long-term adverse effect on his or her ability to carry out normal day-to-day activities.* The list of conditions/impairments which are covered by this definition and further information about rights and benefits available can be found at the Directgov website (**www.direct.gov.uk/en/DisabledPeople/index.htm**).

Each university will have systems and processes in place to support you through your programme. When you have applied to them they should contact you to identify whether you require any reasonable adjustments for your interview. Information about your disability will not be disclosed to anyone without your permission, but it is important to understand that if you choose to limit who may know about your disability, this may limit the support that can be provided both at your interview and once you start your programme.

Once you start your programme the disability team will agree an individual learning plan for you that details the reasonable adjustments you require both in the university and out in practice. You can show this to your lecturers or mentors in practice without revealing your disability if you wish. Additional funding is available to buy equipment and support if you require it and the disability team will help you to apply for this. Examples of some of the reasonable adjustments that might be appropriate are shown in Table 2.1 for some of the more common disabilities seen in nursing.

Student view ... I was really struggling during my first semester, then one of the lecturers said she thought I was dyslexic and referred me to the disability team. The university paid for a test and the lecturer was proved right. After that my world changed. I had additional support to help with my assignments, extra time for exams and a tape recorder to tape classes so I could focus on the sessions rather than trying to make notes that didn't make sense later. I won't say it's been easy, but I wouldn't have got through without all that help and support.

Dyslexia

Dyslexia is one of the most common disabilities seen at university and many now have departments to help support students with specific learning disabilities such as dyslexia. If you have already been diagnosed with dyslexia then the university will require a copy of the report, which must have been undertaken after you were 16 years old. If you have never had an assessment, or you are unsure whether you have dyslexia or not, or your assessment was undertaken before you were 16, then the university can arrange an assessment for you. An excellent range of toolkits for nurses with dyslexia, dyspraxia and dyscalculia can be found on the Royal College of Nursing website (**www.rcn.org.uk**) and will give you an insight into the type of support available to you in practice settings.

Dyslexia	More time to complete exams, provision of a laptop, handouts given in advance, coloured overlays, use of a scribe
Visual impairment	Handouts in preferred format, specialist equipment such as talking thermometers, blood pressure monitors, blood glucose monitors, recorded handovers, note takers, extra time in examinations, flexible shift patterns
Auditory impairment	Amplified stethoscope, handouts given in advance, tape recorder for lectures, British Sign Language interpreter, placements that are smaller/quieter without too much background noise
Mental health difficulties/chronic illness	Flexible work patterns to enable optimum performance, time out to attend hospital appointments

Table 2.1: Examples of reasonable adjustments for disabilities

Lecturer tip ... Check out the websites of the universities you are interested in to see what help and support they can offer you if you have a disability.

I'm not a traditional student: is nursing possible for me?

One of the great things about nursing is that it attracts a diverse range of students and the NMC, employers and universities encourage this. As we said above the average age of student nurses is over 25. Students also enter from a wide range of academic backgrounds, with entry qualifications including A levels, Scottish Highers, Irish leaving certificates, the Access to Nursing Course as well as degrees in other subject areas. Universities are also keen to attract students from diverse ethnic backgrounds to reflect the diversity of the patients and service users they will be caring for. If you are worried about fitting in, try to attend the open days at the universities you are interested in as this will give you the best feel about the diversity of students that you will be studying with and whether a particular university will suit you.

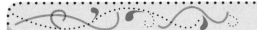

Chapter summary

This chapter should have helped you to consider whether you have got what it takes to study nursing and become a nurse. The focus has been on the skills, attitudes and values which are so important in nursing. The next chapter will look at other entry requirements for getting into nursing.

Further reading

NHS Careers (2011) *Work Experience in the NHS: A toolkit for teachers and work placement organisers.* Available from: **http://www.nhscareers.nhs.uk/media/1487492/Work_experience_in_the_NHS.pdf**

Although aimed at teachers and work placement organisers, this guide provides useful information about gaining work experience in the NHS.

Nursing and Midwifery Council (2015) *The Code: Professional standards of practice and behaviour for nurses and midwives.* London: NMC. Available from: **http://www.nmc-uk.org/Publications/Standards/The-code/Introduction**

The code outlines the expectations of the NMC with regard to your conduct as a professional nurse and will enable you to appreciate what it means to be a registered professional.

Useful websites

Each country in the UK has its own processes for bursaries:

England: **www.nhsbsa.nhs.uk/Students.aspx** which also has a bursary calculator.

Northern Ireland: **www.nursingandmidwiferycareersni.com/bursary.html**

Scotland: **www.saas.gov.uk/full_time/nmsb**

Wales: **www.weds.wales.nhs.uk/funding-support-for-those-taking-nhs-cou**

www.disabilityalliance.org

The Disability Alliance website has a range of publications about your rights if you have a disability, with some specifically for students with a disability.

www.nmc-uk.org/Students/Guidance-for-students

See the section of the Nursing and Midwifery Council website for student nurses for information about what is expected of you as a student.

www.thestudentroom.co.uk

The Student Room has forums and wikis which provide useful information about being a student, nurse, nursing programmes, practice experiences and the different universities that offer nursing programmes.

www.aquestionofcare.org.uk

While not aimed at nurses specifically, this website provides some excellent videos on care services for children, the elderly and people with a learning disability and allows you to undertake a challenge to see if a career in any of these areas is for you.

Chapter 3
Entry requirements

Beattie Dray and Kim Tolley

Chapter aims

The aim of this chapter is to explore the entry requirements for nursing programmes. By the end of this chapter you will be able to:

- appreciate the specific academic entry requirements for nursing degree programmes;
- consider alternative routes into nursing;
- discuss other attributes and values necessary to enhance your application;
- appreciate issues such as widening participation and gaining work experience.

Introduction

If you want to get onto a nursing course, a key consideration is making sure that you have the appropriate academic qualifications. This chapter will consider the various types of educational qualifications that you need for entry to nursing degrees. As well as qualifications, which are essential to be considered for any programme, you need to demonstrate other attributes, such as commitment to a nursing career and your chosen field of nursing. Personal qualities such as being non-judgmental and caring are also essential.

Gaining experience in a healthcare setting is quite difficult, but there may be other ways of experiencing healthcare that Chapter 4 reviews. These are the type of things that any admissions tutor will be looking for on your application form and will help you be shortlisted for an interview.

One of the many positive changes in the ways that nurses are trained and educated is the recognition that many people of all ages and backgrounds have the potential to become excellent nurses. Universities are now seeing increasing numbers of mature students applying for nursing programmes and they are particularly keen to recruit students who are representative of the ethnic diversity of their patients.

The minimum academic entry qualifications

There are various types of minimum entry requirement to degree-level nursing programmes, some examples of which are given below. If you do not have these qualifications you can decide which route would be best to take to achieve them. Many universities also offer nursing courses specifically targeted at entrants who already have degrees, as will be discussed in Chapter 5. These programmes may be at Master's or postgraduate level.

A levels and Scottish Highers

The standard entry tariff acceptable for most nursing programmes is between 240 and 280 UCAS tariff points (although an increasing number are asking for higher than this). This equates to CCC to BBC grades at A level and the equivalent grades at Scottish Highers/Advanced Highers that meet the same UCAS points. Each individual university decides on the UCAS points required and how they can be met and this information is published on the university admissions and UCAS websites (**www.ucas.ac.uk**).

Ideally these qualifications should include evidence of study of a health or science-related subject. Some universities may consider applicants with 200 points at clearing or in other exceptional circumstances, for example when only two A level-equivalent subjects were taken.

If you apply with A levels, your GCSE results will also be considered. All applicants, regardless of what additional qualifications they have, must demonstrate that they have the equivalent of maths and English at GCSE level to a minimum of grade C. Most universities will accept key skills equivalents at level 2 for these. This is a requirement laid down by the Nursing and Midwifery Council.

Access courses

Other qualifications considered include the Quality Assurance Agency-recognised Access courses. Most universities usually require a minimum of 45 credits at level 1 and 15 at level 2. Most say that at least 21 of the level 3 credits must be achieved at merit or distinction. Specific Access courses are designed to give those students who complete them all the skills and knowledge required to be successful when starting nurse education programmes. These are called Access to Nursing and Midwifery courses. For example, they have units on numeracy and literacy, but many now require candidates to already have GCSE maths and English or to study it alongside the Access course. They have other units on science, human biology, sociology and psychology. Such courses are ideal for mature students who have been out of full-time education for a long period, as you can gain your entry requirements for nursing in less than one year. However, these courses are solely academically focused and do not include any work experience. The hours of attendance are also compatible with having part-time work. The best thing to do if you are interested in this route is to contact your local further education college or look at its website for details.

BTEC National Diploma

This must be in a health or science-related subject and passed at merit/distinction level. The most common example is the health and social care qualification. These courses are often taken immediately after school, aged 16 plus. These offer work placement experiences, but do not include maths or English, so you would need to have gained these qualifications at GCSE already.

Overseas qualifications

Most universities will consider non-UK equivalent qualifications, such as degrees, A and O levels. Overseas qualifications are verified by UK NARIC, the national agency responsible for providing information, advice and expert opinion on vocational, academic and professional skills and qualifications from over 180 countries worldwide.

Activity 3.1   *Do I meet the academic entry criteria?*

Look at the UCAS website (**www.ucas.ac.uk**) and identify the universities you are interested in. Note their entry requirements. Now list the different academic qualifications you hold and their grades. The UCAS website provides tariff tables at **www.ucas.com/ how-it-all-works/explore-your-options/entry-requirements/tariff-tables**. You can now shortlist the universities for which your qualifications will be acceptable. If you find you don't have the required entry requirements, don't despair; contact the admission department of those universities whose requirements are closest to the academic qualifications you hold and discuss with them what you need to do to meet their entry requirements.

Accreditation of prior learning

Accreditation of prior learning (APL) is offered by universities to candidates who have prior learning from academic study and/or work experience they wish to claim for. The APL process requires applicants to map previous learning against the programme learning outcomes. There will be a designated APL adviser in the university who is able to consider APL claims from candidates and can advise you how to go about the claim. If this applies to you, it is best to ask the admissions team who it is you need to speak to. Usually the maximum allowance for APL is 50% of the award (Nursing and Midwifery Council, 2010). This means that if you have previously undertaken degree studies or a Foundation degree, for example, in a health-related course, you may be able to claim APL for some of the nursing course and complete it sooner. However, this usually means that you join the course later in the programme and not all students are comfortable with missing elements of the course.

Foundation degrees

These provide a relatively new route into nursing, usually undertaken by healthcare assistants who are funded by their employer to undertake the course. Students who have completed a

Foundation Degree in nursing may be able to APL out of the first year of a nursing degree programme (see the section above).

Additional entry requirements and expectations

In addition to demonstrating you have the relevant academic entry requirements, the universities will also require other evidence that demonstrates your suitability to undertake a nursing degree and become a nurse.

Evidence of recent study

If you are a mature student then many universities will require evidence of academic study within the last five years; however, some universities will be flexible about this. Your personal statement will be important in demonstrating your ability to undertake academic studies if you have been out of the education system for a while.

Non-native speakers

If you do not have the equivalent of GCSE English, usually at grade C, then you will have to undertake an International English Language Testing System (IELTS) test and gain a score of 7.0, or equivalent. If you are studying an Access to Nursing programme this will not be necessary as a key skills English language unit will be included in your course, although many Access courses now require GCSE English.

Mature applicants

If you are a mature candidate who does not meet the traditional requirements for programmes, some universities will consider you on an individual basis depending on relevant work experience. Again, your personal statement will be important in demonstrating why you believe you meet the entry requirements.

Work or voluntary experience

Evidence of experience in a health or social care setting is an excellent way of both enabling you to be sure that a career in nursing is the right one for you and enhancing your application. Paid employment within healthcare settings can be difficult to find, particularly if you are under 18 years old. Voluntary work is much easier to undertake and there are many websites that aim to match your interests with the right sort of volunteering. We will explore the best way to find work or voluntary experience in Chapter 4.

Activity 3.2   *Demonstrating you have the appropriate experience*

If you have never worked in a health or social care setting, whether paid or voluntary work, think about examples in your life where you have used your personal caring qualities. For example, you may have cared for an elderly family member or perhaps you are close to someone who experienced a mental health problem and you supported that person through this period. Write brief notes on this. We will come back to this later when developing your personal statement.

Widening participation

Widening participation aims to improve educational opportunities for everyone regardless of age, gender, ethnic group or disability. All nursing programmes aim to encourage widening participation and so put in place strategies to ensure they are inclusive of all these groups. Widening participation has many advantages in nursing, since the nursing workforce should mirror the patient group that it serves.

Good health and good character

Good health and good character are fundamental to fitness to practise as a nurse or midwife (**www.nmc-uk. org**). Admission to any nursing programme, therefore, is always subject to occupational health screening and Disclosure Barring Service (DBS) checks.

Occupational health checks

You will be required to complete an occupational health form and if you disclose any health conditions or disabilities, the occupational health department may contact you for more information. This may be a simple phone call or they may require you to attend their department for a more detailed assessment. As we discussed in Chapter 2, many students with a disability or health condition successfully apply for and complete a nursing programme. The role of the occupational health department is to ensure that if you are affected by a physical or mental health condition it does not impair your ability to practise safely and effectively without supervision.

DBS checks

The system for checking and monitoring of previous criminal convictions and cautions, etc. changed in 2013 to a new system known as the Disclosure and Barring Service. The new system allows for greater flexibility in terms of how those persons who have previous convictions etc. are managed. Having a previous conviction, caution, etc. does not automatically mean that you cannot enter the nursing profession. The new DBS automatic filtering system means that prospective employers or educational institutions will no longer necessarily see all criminal records, depending on the type and how old they are. Once you have completed the online process, the DBS will issue you with an enhanced disclosure certificate. The new system is also a live system, so you may be expected to pay an annual subscription fee for the service. This does mean that you can access your records as and when required, by other institutions, employers etc.

Student view ... I felt ashamed as I knew that I had a caution on my record, which I received when I was 16 years old for shoplifting. I declared this on my UCAS application form. Before my interview I called the admissions tutor and talked to him about this and how it might affect my application. He said that I had done the most important thing, which was to be honest about it. He asked me for details about the caution and what I had learnt from the experience.

If you have committed an offence in the past you will be provided with the opportunity to explain the specific situation and to discuss what you have learnt from the event and how your circumstances have changed since then.

All universities have a process which reviews such applications, and considers an individual's suitability for a professional course such as nursing. You may be asked for a more detailed statement about the events and will need to demonstrate your appreciation as to why certain criminal offences may raise concerns regarding a candidate's suitability to become a nurse. It is important to have thought these issues through when preparing for your interview. There is more information about this in Chapter 8.

If you have any concerns about this area it is best to discuss them with the admissions tutor at the university prior to submitting your application.

Your personal statement

This is the part of the application form that allows you to 'sell yourself' to your chosen universities. Universities receive hundreds of applications for nursing and, having checked that you meet the entry criteria, the admissions tutor will decide whether to offer you an interview based on the content of your personal statement, so getting this right is crucial. We will look at this in more detail in Chapter 8.

The different routes into nursing

Twenty years ago nursing students used to be primarily white 18-year-olds, straight from school with 'O' (GCSEs) and 'A' levels. There were also very few men – around 5%. Today the situation has altered dramatically. On some programmes over 50% of students are over 30 years of age. The number of men in nursing is slowly increasing and averages 10–14%. Nursing students now come from a wide range of ethnic groups, reflecting the local community they are recruited from and wish to care for.

Below are a few case studies to give you a flavour of the type of people that you could be sitting next to in a classroom when you start nursing and the different routes they have taken to get there. The case studies give the background to applicants and the comments by the admissions tutor who looks carefully at each application before deciding whether applicants meet the entry criteria and should be offered an interview.

Case study: Joan

Joan is 42 years old. She did her A levels 25 years ago and passed three at grades B, C and D. She has O levels in English and maths. Joan has been studying book-keeping over the past two years and has just passed these exams. Joan's children have just left home to go to university and she feels it is an opportunity for her to study learning disability nursing, something she has wanted to do since before she was married, but was unable to start as her husband had a busy job and she had the children to bring up. Joan has worked part-time for the last five years as a carer in the community for people with learning disabilities. She has NVQ level 2.

Comment from admissions tutor
Joan has obviously thought carefully about her move into nursing. She will be considered individually as a mature applicant; she has evidence of recent studying and has excellent work experience of caring with people with learning disabilities.

Case study: Kemi

Kemi is an 18-year-old student who has just received her A level results in biology, sociology and media studies. She was pleased to have gained three B grades. Kemi achieved seven GCSEs, including maths; she had to resit English last year and gained a C grade. She wants to move away from home and has chosen a university 100 miles away. Kemi has been on an open day at the university and has decided to apply for children's nursing. She has been volunteering at her local youth club for the last year for her Gold Duke of Edinburgh award.

Comment from admissions tutor
Kemi has done well in her A levels and has carefully considered her career choice, as she has been to open days and thought about where she would like to study. Her recent volunteering shows that she has the commitment to stay in a role for a lengthy period of time and will be able to relate to younger people in the child field of nursing. We would like a reference from the youth leader outlining her responsibilities to be included with her application.

Case study: Jennifer

Jennifer is a 26-year-old student who is halfway through an Access to Nursing course. Jennifer has one son, aged three, and works two days a week for a private care alarm service answering telephone calls. She likes the contact with people who telephone the call centre when they fall, or are worried about anything. Often she has to call an ambulance or arrange for a carer to visit someone's home. Jennifer is applying for adult nursing as she enjoys the contact with older people.

Comment from admissions tutor

We have a good link with the college that runs Jennifer's Access to Nursing course and take a high proportion of their students on our programme. Jennifer will have to do well on her Access course to gain a place on the programme. Her work experience, although not involving direct care delivery, is extremely relevant, since it is related to health and she has expertise in communicating with people and members of the multidisciplinary team. It also sounds like Jennifer has to use her initiative to deal with challenging situations involving adults, some of whom are elderly. We will explore this at interview with her.

Case study: David

David is 40 years old and has been working in the publishing industry for the last 20 years. David has been studying for an Open University degree in psychology for the past six years, and has just completed the course. He was made redundant six months ago and has taken the opportunity to re-evaluate his career. He has always enjoyed working in a team and is fascinated by health. He is attracted to mental health nursing as some of his degree looked at the impact of society on mental wellbeing. David has been volunteering at his local cancer centre, working on the reception there one day a week.

Comment from admissions tutor

David has evidence of recent study and he is eligible for the two-year postgraduate programme at our university. Knowledge gained on his degree will certainly help him with nursing and is strongly linked to the mental health field. His recent experience at the cancer centre has given him an insight into healthcare and will have made him sure of his decision to change careers.

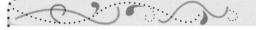

Chapter summary

This chapter has considered the range of entry requirements that are suitable when applying for a nursing programme. One or more of these may apply to you, but if you are unsure, the best way to check is to contact the admissions team at the university that you are interested in. They will be able to give you some individualised information and identify if you have any gaps in your academic or personal experiences to make sure your application meets the requirements of their programme. One of the most important parts of your UCAS application form is the personal statement: it is your opportunity to 'sell yourself' and should make your application stand out from the crowd. We will look at developing your personal statement in Chapter 7.

Useful websites

www.naric.org.uk

NARIC is the national agency that is responsible for providing information, advice and expert opinion on vocational, academic and professional skills and qualifications from over 180 countries worldwide.

www.nmc-uk.org/Students/Good-Health-and-Good-Character-for-students-nurses-and-midwives

The Nursing and Midwifery Council website provides guidance on what it means by good health and good character.

www.ucas.ac.uk

The UCAS website gives details of all the universities that offer nursing programmes and their specific entry requirements.

www.volunteering.org.uk, www.volunteerscotland.net, www.volunteering-wales.net, www.volunteernow.co.uk

These are all organisations that provide information on volunteering opportunities in your local area.

Chapter 4
Work experience and volunteering

Sue Fergy and Kim Tolley

Chapter aims

The aim of this chapter is to explore the work experience and volunteering options for students wanting to enter nursing and to explain why they are so important in the selection process.

By the end of this chapter you will be able to:

- appreciate the reasons why work experience and volunteering are an essential part of getting into nursing;
- understand why being able to demonstrate your values is an essential element of the selection processes for nurses and all healthcare staff;
- discuss the range of work experience and volunteering that is relevant to a nursing application;
- consider the best ways to access work experience and volunteering;
- plan how to get the most from your work experience and volunteering;
- explain how your work experience and volunteering activities can help you demonstrate your values and qualities.

Introduction

Evidence of work experience and volunteering is a vital part of any nursing application. When the university considers your nursing degree application, your personal statement will be assessed and they will look for references to your work experience and volunteering within it. Your work and volunteering experiences can demonstrate one of two things. First, if it is in health or social care, it will show that you have taken the time to really find out about what a career in health entails and whether this is the right career for you. Otherwise, it can show the university that you are able to identify the skills and values you have gained and apply them to the field of nursing that you have chosen to apply for.

The best way to find work experience is to keep an eye on local newspapers and job websites. Remember that it does not have to be paid employment as a healthcare assistant; it can be, for example, working with a charity or as a volunteer receptionist in a hospital or hospice.

Why are values so important in the selection process?

In 2013, Sir Robert Francis published a report, which told the story of the appalling suffering of many hospital patients within a culture of secrecy and defensiveness. The Francis public enquiry focused on one organisation – Mid Staffordshire NHS Foundation Trust – but it showed that many of the failures existed across the range of healthcare settings. The final report made 290 recommendations to be implemented by a range of organisations including universities (Francis, 2013).

One of the report's key recommendations is that staff being recruited into the NHS should be tested to show how their values and behaviours meet those of the NHS. These values can be found in the NHS Constitution, which would be a useful document to look at before your interview, along with the Francis Report. In response to this report, universities and Trusts are now focusing on values-based recruitment which means that they are looking for evidence that the people they are recruiting have the values and the qualities that are important to patients.

For nursing, the Chief Nurse has identified specific values that should be demonstrated by all nurses both as students and when qualified; these are known as the '6Cs':

- care;
- compassion;
- competence;
- commitment;
- communication;
- courage.

You therefore need to show how the work you have undertaken, either as a volunteer or in a paid capacity, can demonstrate how you possess these values.

What do you want from your work experience or voluntary work?

Before you apply it would be a good idea for you to write down some aims for the experience. What do you want to get out of it?

For example, you could include:

- to gain insight into a career in adult/mental health/children's or learning disability nursing;
- to find out what nurses actually do each day;
- to talk to patients about what is important to them;

- to talk to patients and find out why they are in hospital;

- to talk to nurses and other healthcare professionals about their job;

- to talk to nurses and other health professionals about the challenges in their job and what they enjoy most;

- to discuss with nurses and other health professionals what they find stressful in their job roles;

- to see what nurses do that make a difference to the care patients receive.

Looking at the aims we have listed, use these to help you compile your own aims in order of importance. When you are invited to interview you can refer to your list: it shows again that you have thought about this and are keen to access work experience.

Student view ... I managed to get some voluntary work with Mind and I'm glad I did as it really confirmed that mental health nursing was the right career for me. A number of students dropped out after their first placement because they'd had no previous experience and then found mental health nursing wasn't what they expected.

Lecturer view ... Applicants who have had some experience in a health or social care setting are generally better able to demonstrate a more realistic understanding of what nursing is and what skills they will need. I remember one student who had done some voluntary work helping on a holiday camp for young people with learning disabilities. Her understanding of their needs and the shock she felt when she saw the way people responded to them when they took them out told me that here was someone who had both commitment and compassion and would be ideal for learning disability nursing.

The range of work experience

Working in healthcare

Ideally, of course, you will probably prefer to gain work experience, either paid or unpaid, in the field of nursing that you want to apply for. You can search your local healthcare trusts or care homes, for example, for work as a healthcare assistant, or other positions that will give you contact with patients and service users, such as a receptionist or ward administrator or patient services administrator. Many of these jobs do not require you to have experience and they will give you training to undertake the role. If still at school, you may wish to consider taking a year off before applying to university to gain sufficient experience and ensure nursing is the right career for you. If you are lucky you may find that one of your local hospitals is offering one of the new pre-nursing experiences currently being piloted in England.

Pre-nursing experience pilot schemes

In one of the recommendations of the Francis Report (2013) the government asked Health Education England to implement and evaluate a pilot scheme for prospective nurse students to work for up to a year as a healthcare assistant (HCA), to gain care experience and test their values and behaviours of care and compassion. The aim of the pilot is to recruit aspiring student nurses, with no or little experience, into paid HCA posts from September 2013, allowing them to gain caring experience in real jobs, testing to see if they are right for the job and that the job is right for them. Through these pilots, prospective nursing students are on paid placements, providing care for patients now whilst building their own experience and preparing them better for their university courses. You can learn more by visiting Health Education England's website: **http://hee.nhs.uk/work-programmes/ pre-nursing-care-experience-pilots**

Work experience related to healthcare

Many local hospitals run programmes of work experience which will be described on their website. They usually require completion of an application and you will be asked to explain why you want to join the programme. It is important to refer to the fact that you want to become a registered nurse and that this experience will give you an important insight into the profession. You may be asked to attend an interview for this work experience.

However, if gaining relevant work experience is not possible for you, maybe because there are no local vacancies, you may have to compromise and choose another option.

Work experience in alternative areas

There are many jobs which will help you to develop skills that will be useful in nursing. At first glance a job in retail, restaurants, hotels or a pub, for example, may not seem to be relevant when applying to start your career in nursing. But if you are working in these areas or others similar to them you will have direct contact with the public and you will have to use many skills that are very relevant for nursing, e.g. good timekeeping, organisational skills, demonstrating competence (that is, your ability to perform given tasks well), and good communication skills.

Let's use a job in retail to show how the skills that you might use in this type of job can be useful when applying for nursing. If you have worked in retail, tick the skills in Table 4.1 that you use every day to ensure that you do a good job. Otherwise, apply the ideas to your own work experience as many areas are likely to be relevant.

Using Table 4.1 will help you see that you use many very important skills in your job (and can demonstrate at least three of the 6Cs!). Whatever experiences you have, you can demonstrate a wide range of qualities and skills if you think about it. The challenge for you is to:

- ensure that you can link your attributes to a specific field of nursing;
- find ways of showing these attributes during the application process.

Skills	Example of when you use this skill	Tick if you use these in your job
Timekeeping	Ensuring that you arrive promptly and return from your breaks on time.	
Leadership and using your initiative	If there is a spillage on the shop floor, you might organise to clear it up yourself or call the cleaner to do it. You don't just leave it.	
Teaching	Showing others how to do elements of the job role, for example showing new starters how to work a till/card machine.	
Organisational skills	Organising the lunch break rota or calling for assistance when there is a queue building up and you need more help on the tills.	
Stock control	Restocking shelves and displaying food in date order, so that the food with the nearest date is at the front of the display.	
Communication	Dealing with the returns of goods or calmly managing unhappy or angry customers.	
Commitment and reliability	Not letting your colleagues or employer down by missing shifts or always arriving late.	
Negotiating	If you need to take a holiday or change shifts negotiating with your team or your boss.	
Explaining	Explaining to customers where certain items are – or why they are not in stock.	
Information technology	Using IT in stock control or ordering supplies online.	
Telephone skills	Dealing with customer queries on the phone or making calls to customers to organise delivery of their goods.	
Respect and tolerance	Treating all of your customers in a kind and fair manner – regardless of their age, gender, ethnicity, ability to communicate clearly or disability.	

Table 4.1: Skills and their use: an example from retail

This is why your personal statement is so important – it is your first opportunity to demonstrate to the university that you understand what qualities and skills they are looking for in potential nurses – and that you have them.

So, for example, in your retail role you may have stated in Table 4.1 that that you use teaching skills when you show new starters in the shop how to use the tills and also the credit card machine.

To do this part of your role you must also demonstrate patience and the ability to explain things in a way that is understandable to an inexperienced person who may be nervous. You might need to explain how you have done this – by using very simple language and by breaking the task down into small, easy steps so that they can then put the task together and do it competently.

Teaching and explaining are important skills that any nurse needs to be able to demonstrate. For example, a children's nurse may have to use these skills when teaching a newly diagnosed teen-ager about their diabetes and how to give themselves an injection. Or a nurse might have to show an 8-year-old with asthma how to use an inhaler. To do this as a children's nurse you need to be able to use your teaching skills, in a patient manner, using language that does not 'talk down' to the child. You would also need to be able to explain these techniques to the child or young person in a way that is easy to understand, perhaps by breaking it down into small steps – and repeat them if the child does not understand immediately.

Another example of how your work experience may have helped you develop a strong work ethic is that you may have identified that you use your timekeeping skills to ensure that you arrive for your shift five minutes before it starts to prepare yourself, and arrive back from breaks on time. To do this you have to be organised, get up on time and plan your time well, including the journey to work.

These are all vital skills for registered nurses. After all it would not be fair – or professional – for a nurse to be late for their shift. Not only is it uncaring for those who have been working, but it could mean that you miss the handover of essential information.

You may have identified communication as a skill you have developed. If you work in a job that deals directly with the public you may have encountered people who are angry, stressed or dissatisfied with the service they have been provided. It is important that you treat each customer politely and with respect using the 'customer is always right' philosophy. When doing this you need to be clear and assertive and deal with situations calmly and fairly under pressure – especially if there is queue of other customers waiting. Providing an example of how you managed a difficult situation can demon-strate effective use of your communication skills. The same skills can be used in nursing. For exam-ple, worried visitors who come to the ward may ask to see the nurse in charge to find out how their relative is and want to talk to them instantly. It is important to treat visitors politely, but you may need to explain that the nurse in charge is busy at the moment, doing the medicines round and that the nurse will come and see them when the round is finished. It is essential that you communicate with the relatives politely and reassure them that you will pass on their message. It is also important that you relay the message to the nurse in charge at the appropriate time.

We have given you a few examples of how the skills and values you currently use at work can be applied to your future career in nursing. Now it is up to you to work out how this can be applied to your current job role.

To help your thinking on this topic, most organisations have a mission statement or a philosophy, which spells out their values; find out what values your organisation considers to be important.

For example, on their website, Tesco states that it aims to be *responsible, fair and honest*. The St John Ambulance charity explains on its website that it aims to achieve its *charitable mission in responsible ways that benefit all of those we work with and serve . . . we want to care for people directly; we want to ensure that their lives and their environment are as healthy and positive as possible.*

Refer back to the values of nursing (the NHS and the 6Cs). What similarities are there between the values of the NHS and the organisation you have been working in? How have you developed these skills and values from spending time in your organisation?

In a copy of Table 4.2 list the skills you have identified as ones you use at work in your current role and in the next column state how they can be applied to nursing and more specifically your chosen field of nursing.

Skills and values you use in your current role	Examples of how these skills can be used in nursing and in your chosen field

Table 4.2: Skills and their use: your current role and relevance to nursing

These examples in Table 4.2 will be ones you can refer to in your personal statement for your UCAS application.

Voluntary work

If you cannot get paid employment it shows great commitment and determination to undertake an unpaid, voluntary role.

There is a range of volunteer jobs, for example:

- befriending people in nursing homes;
- working in a charity shop;
- working on an information desk or as a hostess guiding people round a hospital;
- driving people to hospital appointments;
- acting as family link volunteer;
- participating as a play worker;
- working in visitor centres in prisons;
- managing fund raising for a charity or good cause;

- managing a tea bar/trolley;
- helping at a soup kitchen or food bank;
- sharing your talents as a musician, entertainer or performer;
- volunteering overseas – e.g. working in an orphanage or school.

Experience in any one of these roles should be described in your personal statement – with you clearly identifying the link between what you have *done* and what you have *learnt* from it or how it has helped you *develop* your skills, knowledge and values. Voluntary work demonstrates that you want to make a positive difference to people's lives and is an attribute which is looked for in nurses.

Using the same techniques we discussed earlier, identify the ways your voluntary work links with nursing.

Case study

Josie does voluntary work. Each Saturday morning, she works at her local learning disability charity shop. She takes donations that arrive and then sorts out the stock into goods that can be sold, and goods that need to be moved to the charity's furniture store. She also works on the tills and helps cover the changing rooms. Sometimes, Josie works alongside other volunteers, some of whom have learning disabilities, and she has learnt some useful lessons about effective communication with them.

In her personal statement Josie says:

> *For the past seven months, I have volunteered at my local charity shop each Saturday morning. I enjoy taking the donations from the public and getting them signed up for Gift Aid donations. This involves categorising their donations and using the computer. In addition, I have experience of working in a team with people who have learning disabilities. At first this was not very comfortable for me, but I looked up Mencap's guidelines for talking with people with learning disabilities and realised I needed to adapt – to talk on a one-to-one basis, to talk more slowly, not to hurry people up and to make good eye contact. These skills are relevant to nursing and in particular the learning disability field.*

Josie is demonstrating examples of her care, competence, compassion and communication.

You may have been involved with volunteering for an award, such as the Duke of Edinburgh Award scheme where you had to volunteer for a period of time. You can also mention this in your personal statement, describing how the experience helped you develop your teamwork skills, together with your commitment, stamina and resilience.

Use contacts through your family and friends to gain access to volunteer work, for example in a youth club, or playgroup at church at which you might volunteer.

Most NHS Trust websites have specific areas for volunteers. Searching on your local hospitals website is a good place to start, but if they don't have anything that attracts you, you need to be willing to look further afield. Again this shows commitment (one of the 6Cs), initiative and a willingness to work hard to gain access to a scheme that would suit your needs and give you an insight into healthcare.

If you have really good IT skills, you might offer your services to a charity to upgrade their website, for example, or help them with installing upgraded software or building a database.

In your local area there will be a volunteer agency, which is a good starting point if you are unsure what volunteering opportunities are available in your community. Staff there will try to direct you to something that meets your needs in terms of the amount of time you can devote to volunteering, and voluntary experiences which will help to prepare you for a nursing career. When you contact them, do explain that your long-term goal is to become a registered nurse.

Your interview for work experience or voluntary work

You will probably be asked to attend an interview for any work experience scheme, and you will find Chapter 8 really useful in preparing for this interview. Take your preparation for the interview seriously. It will be very good practice for your interview at university. Similar qualities and skills will be looked for in both interviews.

How to get the most from your work experience

So, now that you have found work experience, it is vital that you both enjoy it and gain as much as possible from it. You need to revisit the aims that you wrote for yourself at the beginning of this chapter.

Remind yourself that this work experience is a step towards reaching your goal to become a registered nurse – keep that goal in sight!

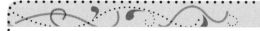

Chapter summary

This chapter has explained the importance of work and voluntary experiences in helping you demonstrate that you have the values and skills required to become a registered nurse. We have looked at the range of opportunities available and helped you to appreciate the relevance of your work experience, even if it is unrelated to healthcare. Key to success is to always keep your aim of getting into nursing in sight, and see every opportunity as a way to help you to access your future career choice.

Useful websites

The Prince's Trust offers help with work experience: **www.princes-trust.org.uk/need_help/courses/get_into.aspx**

Prospect: work experience if you already have a degree: **www.prospects.ac.uk/jobs_and_work_experience.htm**

Volunteering England and Do it! provide access to volunteering opportunities in healthcare settings. A useful place to look for volunteering opportunities in your local area: **www.volunteering.org.uk**

Volunteer Northern Ireland: www.volunteernow.co.uk

Volunteer Scotland: www.volunteerscotland.net

Volunteer Wales: **www.volunteering-wales.net**

NHS Careers page, advising on work experience and volunteering opportunities: **http://nursing.nhscareers.nhs.uk/skills/workexperience**

NHS Careers YouTube channel – view all the NHS Careers videos on the NHS Careers YouTube channel.

Step into the NHS: a website which focuses on supporting younger people to enter the NHS: **www.stepintothenhs.nhs.uk/work-experience.aspx**

NHS Constitution: http://hee.nhs.uk/about/nhs-constitution

The Chief Nurse's 6 'C's: www.england.nhs.uk/wp-content/uploads/2012/12/6c-a5-leaflet.pdf

Chapter 5
What is involved in undertaking a nursing course?

Kim Tolley and Maggie Davenport

Chapter aims

The aim of this chapter is to explore what is involved in studying for a nursing qualification. By the end of the chapter you will be able to:

- appreciate what undertaking a nursing degree entails;
- appreciate the challenges of undertaking a postgraduate pre-registration nursing course;
- understand how nursing programmes are organised;
- identify the differences between nursing degree programmes and other programmes at university;
- consider some of the practicalities of undertaking a nursing course, such as attendance, professional behaviour and placement learning opportunities.

Introduction

For you to achieve your goal of becoming a registered nurse you need to undertake a nursing programme at a higher education institute (HEI). HEIs are predominantly universities, but may be other organisations given degree-awarding powers and which are validated (given permission) to run pre-registration nursing programmes by the Nursing and Midwifery Council (NMC). Part of the application process, which will be considered in Chapter 7, is for you to choose the right university for you. In order to do this you need to understand the different types of programme available, so that you can find one that suits your needs and individual requirements. Each pre-registration nursing programme is different, but they must all meet the *Standards for Pre-registration Nursing Education* required by the NMC (Nursing and Midwifery Council, 2010) which set out the learning outcomes to be achieved, key content and hours of theory and practice as well as other aspects of the programme. Individual universities then work with staff from their local health and social care providers and also the people who use these services (service users) to write their own programme to meet the standards and their local healthcare needs. This means that, while there will be many similarities between the programmes run by each university, there will also be differences and these are what may help you in deciding the best university for you, as we discussed in Chapter 3.

The NMC's aim for a graduate programme

The NMC states that:

> *Our standards aim to enable nurses to give and support high quality care in rapidly changing*
> *environments. They reflect how future services are likely to be delivered, acknowledge future*
> *public health priorities and address the challenges of long-term conditions, an ageing*
> *population, and providing more care outside hospitals. Nurses must be equipped to lead,*
> *delegate, supervise and challenge other nurses and healthcare professionals. They must be able*
> *to develop practice, and promote and sustain change. As graduates they must be able to think*
> *analytically, use problem-solving approaches and evidence in decision-making, keep up with*
> *technical advances and meet future expectations.*
> (Nursing and Midwifery Council, 2010, pp4–5)

Each university goes through a rigorous process to ensure its programmes meet the NMC standards and also the standards of the university; this process is called approval. The NMC ensures that all universities gain approval for their programme every five years to make sure that programmes are always updated and meet the needs of patients and healthcare providers.

Types of nursing degree programme

Nursing has moved to being an all-graduate profession in the UK since 2013. Before then the majority of nursing students studied to diploma level and before that at certificate level. There have always been degree programmes; however the numbers remained relatively small until 2013. The move from a certificate to a diploma and then to a degree programme means that the entry criteria and programme content have changed significantly and this chapter will review what some of these changes mean to you now that you are applying for such a course. Many qualified nurses will have studied at these different levels and many are choosing to 'top up' their diploma to a degree at a later date.

There are four main types of programme:

1. Three- or four-year pre-registration degree programmes leading to a BSc or BSc with honours.

2. Programmes for students who are already graduates and whose degrees are in a health-related subject. Usually, these programmes can be completed in less than three years. These are sometimes called 'accelerated' programmes, 'graduate entry' programmes, 'graduate diplomas' or 'postgraduate' programmes and lead to a postgraduate diploma (PgDip) or Master's qualification as well as registration as a nurse. Most universities now run these courses.

3. Programmes leading to a degree and registration in two fields of nursing, e.g. registered nurse: adult and child health. These are usually four years long.

4. MSc pre-registration nursing courses that use accreditation of prior learning to reduce the time spent at university and in clinical practice. Only a small number of universities offer this route into nursing.

Most programmes are full-time, but some universities offer a part-time route, which can take up to five years.

If you do not meet the entry criteria for any of the above programmes you may decide to do a Foundation course. These courses offer you the opportunity to directly progress into a nursing course if you gain a certain grade. These courses have been designed with healthcare providers, to develop the necessary skills and knowledge for you to progress into nursing. They are also an entry point into other healthcare professions, such as midwifery, occupational therapy and physiotherapy.

Certain elements are common to all NMC approved nursing programmes. For example, they must all ensure that the student nurse completes 2300 hours of theoretical content and 2300 hours of practice learning opportunities and are assessed in both theory and practice.

Lecturer tip ... It is important for prospective student nurses to realise that any nursing course is a combination of theory and practice. This is where it differs from many other degree programmes and this can mean that juggling both these elements is exciting and never dull, but can be challenging.

Learning with and from other students

In previous chapters we have discussed how much of a nurse's time is spent working in a varied team of healthcare professionals. Some of your classes will be with nursing students who are studying your chosen field, but some will be with a combination of students from other fields. This is a real bonus as it means that you will mix with a range of people who have experience of and are interested in different areas of nursing. This adds to your breadth of knowledge about nursing.

The NMC also requires that programmes provide opportunities for students to share learning with others in related health and social care fields. This will enhance interprofessional working and collaboration in practice. Specific arrangements may be agreed for shared learning among medical, physiotherapy, radiography, midwifery and social work students. This may be something that attracts you to a particular programme and the opportunities available to meet with other healthcare students is certainly something to ask about when you go to the open days or for your interview.

Student tip ... Choosing a university which also runs programmes for other healthcare professionals is a real positive. We had a session last week with a mix of medical, nursing, clinical physiology, radiography and social work students. It was so powerful when we looked at professionalism and found that we all had a common goal: that we all were working to benefit people's care experiences. We shared what we were afraid of in our jobs and it turned out that a lot of us were scared of dealing with death and dying. I realised that if I was dealing with such a situation in practice the medical students and the radiographer would feel as anxious as I would be and that we needed to support each other.

The course plan

In many universities, the academic year is divided into two semesters and each semester you will study a number of modules. These modules will cover a range of content, including normal and altered physiology, communication skills, ethics, the nursing care of patients with a range of health conditions, health education and promotion, research and evidence-based practice and management skills, to name but a few. University websites should give you more details of the content they cover.

Sept	Oct	Nov	Dec	Jan	Feb	Mar	Apr	May	Jun	Jul	Aug
	Theory		Practice	H	Theory		Practice	H	Theory		Practice		Hols
Sept	**Oct**	**Nov**	**Dec**	**Jan**	**Feb**	**Mar**	**Apr**	**May**	**Jun**	**Jul**	**Aug**
H	Theory			H	Practice		Theory	H	Theory		Practice		Hols
Sept	**Oct**	**Nov**	**Dec**	**Jan**	**Feb**	**Mar**	**Apr**	**May**	**Jun**	**Jul**	**Aug**
H	Theory	Practice		H	Practice	Theory		H	Practice			Hols

Figure 5.1 Sample programme plan. Theory, weeks in university; Practice, weeks in practice settings; H/Hols, holidays.

Figure 5.1 shows a sample programme plan to give you a flavour of a typical nursing degree programme. This plan shows that during each year you will have a certain number of weeks of theory and clinical placements.

If you compare the programme plan with that of a friend who is doing a degree in another subject you will find that there are very obvious differences.

1. There are fewer theory weeks than your friend has and the theory weeks will often mean full days of study, between 9 a.m. and 5 p.m. This is planned to ensure that you meet the required number of hours to complete your programme.

2. Holiday time may be less than for other degrees. This is because programmes leading to registration as a nurse must include 2300 hours of practice learning opportunities and to fit this into your degree studies inevitably means less time for annual leave. In some universities you may find that you are required to spend the summer on placements. This can be very difficult as your friends and family may have longer holidays and you might need to plan for this.

3. There are scheduled weeks for learning in practice settings. This is the main difference from other programmes as half of your leaning is undertaken in practice. This is often one of the attractive elements of nursing programmes, since, unlike many other degrees or postgraduate programmes nursing is practice-focused. You will be allocated practice learning opportunities in a variety of settings, as described in Chapter 1, and some programmes may also offer electives, in which you can choose where you wish to go to gain some of your practice experience during one of your placement periods. This may be either abroad or elsewhere in the UK.

4. The number of reading weeks or class-free days may be less. Again this is to ensure the programme has the hours of theory required by the NMC and as a result it is a more intense programme than many other degrees or postgraduate programmes

5. At the end of the programme, a designated person in the university has to declare to the NMC that you have completed 2300 hours in theory and 2300 hours in practice. As a consequence your attendance on the programme in theory and out in practice will be monitored in a variety of ways, such as registers and time sheets. Any missed time needs to be made up, for example through extra study or extra hours in the next placement and this can place additional demands on you. If at the end of the programme you have not completed the required number of hours you will need to undertake these through extra time in practice or demonstrating how you made up missed theory time and this may delay your completion of the programme. This often comes as a surprise to students and so monitoring your own hours will ensure that you are fully aware how much time you have completed and whether you will need to put in extra hours along the way so that you can complete on time.

Lecturer tip ... We all have unplanned events in our life from time to time and if something like this happens to you then the most important thing is for you to discuss it with your personal tutor and keep in touch with the university.

Student tip . . . Last month my sister suddenly became ill and was admitted to a psychiatric unit. She has a seven-year-old daughter, who I had to look after. She came to stay with me and I had to take her to school and pick her up at the end of the day. I was worried how I would cope as I was at university and some of the sessions started at 9 a.m. and went on to 5 p.m. I spoke to my personal tutor and we looked at the timetables for the next two weeks to work out how I could juggle things to cope.

I had to miss a few sessions, but we discussed how I would keep up using the material on the virtual learning environment. I was also able to ask another mother to pick my niece up from school on the days when I had sessions which could not be missed. My sister was still unwell and in hospital when I went onto placement. By that time my brother came to help and stayed with me when I was on an early shift so that he could take my niece to school in the morning.

It was a very stressful time. I wanted to be there for my sister, but did not want to jeopardise my position on the course. In the end I also had to get an extension for the essay that was due in, but again my personal tutor helped me to negotiate this. I learnt that it is imperative to keep the university informed as they will do everything they can to help you. (Jennifer, a student nurse)

All programmes have progression points, meaning that you have to pass everything in year 1 to move to year 2, and so on. The whole programme is designed to enable you to progress in a seamless fashion. There are also certain time scales that have to be met on your course that are specified by the NMC. For example you have to complete year 1 of the course 12 weeks into year 2, this is often called the '12 week rule'.

Lecturer tip . . . At your selection day it is a good idea to ask for a mock timetable that will enable you to see how the programme is organised from day to day. Are there several long days or a series of short days? Does teaching occur in the evenings? Knowing this will help you decide how you may need to organise your life to meet the demands of the programme.

Approaches to teaching and learning

A variety of teaching and learning methods will be used during your nursing programme. Using a range makes the teaching more interesting and stimulating. The following are some of the approaches that are commonly used.

- Reflective activities: you might be asked to reflect on a situation from your practice experiences and consider what you have learnt from this and how that will influence your future practice.

- Lead lectures and seminars: often a topic is presented as a lead lecture for the whole of your group. For example, you could have a session on mental health issues, such as depression or schizophrenia. This could be followed by a seminar, in a smaller group. This seminar will give you more of an opportunity to ask questions and clarify issues, such as asking how depression differs in the elderly or adolescent population.

- Patient scenarios: these are scenarios based on real-life examples and are used to enable you to apply some of the theoretical learning to practice. Some sample scenarios follow.

Patient scenarios

Mrs Elsie Jones is a 72-year-old widow, who lives on her own in a third-floor block of flats. She had a fall three weeks ago and fractured her femur.

Janet is a seven-year-old who has been admitted to the day surgery unit for a tonsillectomy.

June is a 62-year-old retired schoolteacher who has been in the mental health unit for three weeks with depression.

Lloyd is a 16-year-old young man with Down's syndrome. He has been in hospital with a chest infection.

What preparations will you need to make for each of these patients to go home?

- Patient narratives: service users contribute to sessions, providing a unique and real-life overview of their experiences of healthcare. These are very powerful sessions and they give you the opportunity to hear at first-hand what their journey through healthcare is actually like.

- Simulations and skills demonstrations: these sessions give you the opportunity to be taught clinical skills in a safe setting, called skills laboratories or simulation centres. You will be given the opportunity to practise nursing skills on each other, role players and manikins. This will help you to perfect your practical techniques before going out to practise them in the real world. The laboratories recreate the facilities of a hospital ward or community setting where you can practise skills such as moving and handling, giving injections and basic life support. You may also have the opportunity to learn a range of skills through role play with patients or service users and share learning with student doctors and other healthcare students. The skills laboratories are a place where you can make mistakes in a safe and supportive environment. Time spent undertaking simulated learning can also count towards your time in practice settings.

- Action learning sets: these involve you working in small groups, initially with a lecturer as a facilitator, but as you progress through the course you may be expected to facilitate these groups yourself. In the group you will work out solutions to problems or patient scenarios and everyone will be given a role to contribute. For example, you could look at one of the scenarios discussed above and discuss research on depression or chest infections.

- Virtual learning activities: each university will have a virtual learning area on the internet containing the modules you are studying with additional content and activities to assist your learning. Lecturers may add notes to the area before or after sessions and provide a variety of quizzes, tests, reading lists or other activities to engage in. It is important to keep up to date with these activities as they are designed to support your learning.

Assessment strategies

Your nursing degree programmes will include a variety of assessments. You will have experienced some of these in your previous studies (e.g. exams and essays), but some may be new, e.g. case studies, clinical skills examinations, blogs and presentations. Most assessments will ask you to apply what you have learnt to your experiences in nursing practice. The assessments are specifically designed to assess the learning outcomes of the programme and ensure that by the end of the course you have the necessary skills, knowledge and attitudes to register as a nurse.

Theoretical assessment

There are two types of assessment: formative and summative. Formative assessments provide you with feedback to enable you to make improvements prior to submitting or taking the summative assessment. Summative theoretical assessments are those which are graded, which you must pass to progress through the programme and which will be linked to specific modules.

> *Student tip* . . . Start your assignments early; that way if you find you are struggling you have time to seek help.

Assessment of practice

Half of your programme is spent in practice settings and so 50% of your assessments will be practice-focused. There are two types of practice assessments: those that take place in the university, and those out in practice settings.

In the university, skills are tested in clinical skills examinations. These can be quite nerve-wracking as you will be watched performing skills which you will need to be competent at when you are in clinical practice, such as:

- temperature, pulse and blood pressure monitoring;
- moving and handling;
- first aid;
- communication;
- basic life support.

These skills are fundamental to all fields of nursing.

Student tip . . . I found my clinical skills assessments quite stressful, but I was so proud when I passed them as it gave me confidence when I was on placement. Finding time to practise in the skills laboratory in advance of the assessment really helped me.

The other part of your practice assessment is completed whilst you are out in practice and undertaken by a qualified nurse mentor who will assess you on your competence in practice. You will be allocated a new nurse mentor each time you go out to practice and this person is responsible for facilitating and supporting your learning and for assessing your level of competence. All mentors undertake a programme to prepare them for their role and are required to attend an annual update on mentorship to ensure that they can continue to support you effectively.

Your mentor will be available to you for at least 40% of your time on placement and will be aware of the requirements of your programme and your practice assessment document. The mentor will complete this with you at the end of each placement and sign to confirm that you are at the required competency level. Your assessment of competence in practice carries equal weighting with your theory assignments and you will be required to pass each practice assessment in order to complete the programme. This is important as a registered nurse must have both the academic knowledge and the practical skills to function competently in their role.

Managing study time

A major challenge for student nurses is managing the hours of studying and preparation for assessments required when they are also spending time out in practice undertaking a variety of shifts. This is even more of a challenge if you have family commitments and if you do, you will need to be far more organised than the other students, as you will not have the same amount of free time available to you. Access to the internet will be crucial to you, as this will provide you with access to the university learning resources when you do have free time. It is likely that you will be asked at interview how you will manage your time on the course so take time to consider this.

Additional expectations of student nurses

There are a number of other areas where a nursing degree/postgraduate diploma differs from a more traditional non-professional degree route.

Professional behaviour

As a nursing student you are subject to expectations about your behaviour, which other students at university are not. These expectations relate to your time in the university, out in practice and in your personal life.

Activity 5.1   *Professional behaviour*

Take a look at the NMC's guidance on professional conduct for students on their website (**www.nmc-uk.org/Students/Good-Health-and-Good-Character-for-students-nurses-and-midwives**) and consider what this might mean to how you will need to conduct yourself during the programme.

You will be required to demonstrate at your interview an appreciation of what will be expected of you as a nurse, so if you refer to this guidance you are likely to impress your interviewers.

You may be asked to sign a student contract or learning agreement to confirm that you understand the expectations the university and the NMC have of you during your programme. It is important to realise that, unlike other students, your conduct as a student and in your personal life could have an impact on your ability to complete the programme. This may be daunting, but it is important that you are aware that a nursing degree asks a lot more of you than a degree that doesn't lead to a professional career. A real-life case study illustrates this.

Case study

George is in the second year of his nursing programme and was out with a group of his friends at the local pub. He got involved in a fight with a few others and was arrested. The police issued him with a caution, which he accepted. George did not think to inform his lecturers at university for six months. He told them after a lecture on professionalism when the lecturer talked about what to do if you received a caution. George

---

continued . . .

was then referred to the university Fitness to Practise panel. George was upset and very worried. He realised that he should not have got involved in the trouble and he should have told the university straight away about his caution. He was aware that he was putting himself at risk of being discontinued from the course as one of the vital parts of being a professional was to be honest and not get into trouble with the police.

There are several issues here for George. First, he was involved in a fight and so exhibiting violent behaviour that would raise concerns about his suitability to become a nurse, as nursing involves caring for vulnerable people. Second, he failed to inform the university immediately (this is a requirement by all universities and the NMC). Lastly, this might have been reported in the local press, bringing the university and nursing into disrepute. At the end of the programme the university has to sign a declaration of good character, which states that you are capable of safe and effective practice as a nurse, and therefore, you must always keep the university informed about issues that might reflect poorly on your good character.

Caution should also be taken when using social networking sites. The NMC provides guidance on its website about their use which is worth reading as you may need to reconsider how you use social media. It is vital to consider the history that you have on social media and the image that you portray. In years to come when you are applying for jobs as a registered nurse recruiters may look at your social media history. It would be a good idea now to consider your social media accounts, what are the privacy settings and who can see what you have written? Even more importantly, what would any future patient think of your profile? You will have more information on this when you start the nursing programme.

Diversity and inclusivity

University students, staff, practice colleagues, patients and service users come from a wide diversity of backgrounds. This variety of cultures is to be valued and welcomed. As nurses we must be able to provide nursing care for patients and service users, which includes touching people and sometimes providing intimate care irrespective of age, gender, culture, beliefs, disability or disease. Nurses must also be honest, polite and respectful to everyone they encounter whilst undertaking the programme and once qualified.

Also, to ensure adequate communication and accurate identification, it is important to expose your face fully to patients, colleagues and staff in all practice and teaching settings. This is vital for the purposes of recognition and clear communication for patients and service users. If you have any concerns about this you need to discuss them at your selection day.

Dress code

Nurses must look professional, whether they wear uniform or not; this is one way to help patients and service users feel confident in us and trust us. If it looks as though we cannot care for ourselves, why should patients trust us to care for them? For adult and children's nursing, uniform is usually worn. The university usually supplies your uniform, but it is your responsibility to keep it clean and make sure that it is worn correctly each day.

For mental health and learning disability nursing a uniform is not normally worn; however you still need to be presented in a professional manner. This means that you should not wear jeans or T-shirts with logos on and should present yourself each day for placement looking clean and smart.

Comfortable shoes are essential as in whatever field of nursing you are about to follow you will be doing quite a lot of walking. As soon as you get a place on a programme you should buy at least one pair of good, black, flat lace-up shoes. Then it is vital to wear them in and make sure that they are comfortable.

Certain rules apply whatever field of nursing you are about to study:

- You are not allowed to have in place any piercings, except for one set of stud earrings.
- Only wear one plain ring.
- Your hair must be kept tidy and for most clinical placements worn above the collar.

All universities will have a dress code or uniform policy for student nurses and you will be provided with this when you start.

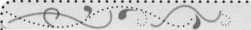

Chapter summary

This chapter has considered the different types of programme that are available to you and how they are run. So far you may have thought that your main aim is to secure a place on a nursing course, but having read this chapter you will see that a nursing course is far more demanding than many other university courses and so you need to consider the best university and programme for your needs. To do this you need to find out as much as you can about each programme and university. In Chapter 7 we will explore how to choose the right university for you, but first you need to be sure you choose the right field of nursing: this is the subject of Chapter 6. It provides you with an overview of the parts of any nursing programme, related to assessments, teaching methods and ways in which you should present yourself.

Further reading

Siviter, B (2013) *The Student Nurse Handbook*, 3rd edition. Edinburgh: Balliere Tindall.
A really good overview of student life in nursing with excellent hints and tips.

Useful website

www.nmc-uk.org/Nurses-and-midwives/Advice-by-topic/A/Advice/Social-networking-sites
Guidance from the NMC on the use of social networking sites for nurses, midwives and nursing students.

Chapter 6
Choosing the right field of nursing

Maggie Davenport, Rosi Castle, Mary Brady, Penny Smith and Martyn Keen

Chapter aims

The aim of this chapter is to introduce you to the four fields of nursing. By the end of the chapter you will be able to:

- appreciate the differences between the four fields of nursing;
- demonstrate an insight into the type of work nurses undertake in each field;
- identify what previous work or voluntary experiences may help support your personal statement for your chosen field;
- give a rationale as to why you have chosen your field of nursing.

Introduction

When completing your UCAS application for a nursing degree you will find that you cannot simply select 'nursing' but have to choose which field of nursing you are interested in as each field will have a different code. There are several reasons for this. Universities are commissioned to recruit a specific number of students for each field of practice; therefore they need to be sure they have selected the appropriate numbers of each field before the course starts. The largest numbers of places are in adult nursing, usually followed by mental health nursing and child health, with learning disabilities usually the smallest group.

The other reason, and most important for you, is that universities want to be sure that the people they select for a specific field are genuinely interested in that field, which means that you must have a clear understanding of what nursing in that field encompasses. It is not always possible to change field once you have started.

Lecturer tip . . . Your personal statement should clearly indicate what field of nursing you are applying for and what qualities you possess that are particularly suitable for your chosen field. A good statement is essential if you want to be offered an interview.

If you are already sure of your chosen field, use this chapter to improve your knowledge and understanding in preparation for writing your personal statement and that all-important selection day. If you are unsure, try Activity 6.1 before reading on.

Activity 6.1   *Which field of practice would be right for me?*

If you are unsure which field of practice might suit you, NHS Careers has a website with a brief personality questionnaire that you may find helpful. Go to **http://nursing.nhscareers.nhs.uk/careers/personality_quiz**; complete the quiz and note what it says about your suitability for nursing and the field(s) of nursing that might suit you best.

Adult nursing

Adult nursing is a person-centred profession with the primary aim of *promoting the well-being and social inclusion of all people through improving or maintaining physical and mental health* (Department of Health, 2010). It is now underpinned by the '6Cs' which are values that all nurses should adhere to in their practice (Chief Nursing Officer and DH Chief Nursing Advisor, 2012): competence, courage, care, communication, compassion and commitment. Using these values, adult nurses provide care for people with a variety of health and social care needs, both simple and complex, and across different age groups. You will be expected to have an understanding of all the fields of nursing as you will, at times, come into contact with people with both a physical illness and mental health problems or a learning disability and will come into contact with children in some departments, such as Accident and Emergency, or when working with families.

Adult nurses need to acquire the knowledge, skills and attitudes that will enable them to provide nursing care in a variety of settings for individuals with diverse levels of complex needs and dependency. All individuals, whether they have mental or physical health problems or a learning disability, have a right to a full and active life. The adult nurse is pivotal in helping individuals and their families or carers in achieving the lifestyles that are important to them. This enables individuals to maintain a quality of life that is right for them.

The adult nurse is viewed as a compassionate professional who will promote health and provide skilled nursing care, creating new partnerships and developing with all patients and service users a therapeutic relationship in each stage of their healthcare journey, including end-of-life care. This relationship ensures that patients are empowered to make choices and maximise their health and wellbeing, and actively engage with people making choices about their health and care and supporting 'no decision about me without me' (DOH, 2012).

Adult nurses collaborate with a variety of health and social care professionals to enhance the experience of patients and to ensure quality outcomes of care. It is often the adult nurse who co-ordinates interprofessional working, so you will need to understand other roles within health and social care; this will also help you consider creative and innovative solutions to clinical issues. Some of these professions are shown in Table 6.1.

The role of the nurse is continually changing as we adapt to a dynamic health environment; people live longer and are more likely to have multiple and complex needs. Nurses are required to learn new skills and take on more responsibilities, and they need to be well informed and flexible in order to respond to those changes. The adult nurse will provide nursing expertise in a wide range of organisations, including the NHS, community, local authorities, independent and voluntary sectors.

General practitioner	District nurse	Social worker
Medical/surgical/ dementia consultant	Clinical nurse specialist – endocrinology/ oncology/orthopaedics/urology/HIV	Speech and language therapist
Health visitor	Occupational therapist	Dietician
Community matron	Mental health or learning disability nurses	Physiotherapist
Acute matron	Pharmacist	Psychiatrist

Table 6.1: Who do adult nurses work with?

What experience is relevant to adult nursing?

Of the four fields, gaining experience in adult nursing is possibly the easiest. Paid work or voluntary experience is equally valuable. Possible areas to consider are:

- voluntary work such as St John Ambulance or British Red Cross;
- working within a residential or care home;
- charity work, such as with Age UK;
- work experience in a hospital, local authority, walk-in centre or within a care team setting in the community;
- healthcare assistant work within a hospital ward or adult community care team;
- caring for elderly relatives.

What qualities do patients and their families see as important for an adult nurse?

The Nursing and Midwifery Council (2010) states:

Adult nurses who acquire the knowledge, skills and behaviours that meet our standards will be equipped to meet these present and future challenges, improve health and wellbeing and drive up standards and quality, working in a range of roles including practitioner, educator, leader and researcher. As autonomous practitioners, nurses will provide essential care to a very high standard and provide complex care using the best available evidence and technology where appropriate.

Through your training you will meet a wide variety of people, so that as a qualified nurse you have the ability to be patient and flexible in your approach, taking into account the diversity of people, their carers and families requiring healthcare.

Carer view . . . Student adult nurses need to have the core values that come with being a professional nurse. They need to look at how they present themselves and how this affects the way they treat people.

It is important that the healthcare team appreciate the views and opinions of patients and their carers/families; the nurse is their advocate wherever necessary. Nurses will also be expected to help people make informed decisions by giving them information that is appropriate to their needs and their situation.

In order to provide appropriate and effective care, nurses must reflect on their knowledge and skills to ensure that these are based on strong evidence and that they have the skills to critically appraise research findings which may influence patients'/service users' care prior to and during their implementation (Standing, 2014).

Nurses' views . . . Adult nursing has changed significantly in the last few years. The majority of patients in hospitals are elderly, acutely ill with multiple health problems and many also have dementia. This means adult nurses in hospitals need to be able to survive in a very busy environment with patients constantly being admitted and discharged.

Being an adult nurse gives you so much scope to advance your career with many students going straight into the community for their first post or deciding to work abroad.

Children and young people's nursing

Children and young people's nursing spans the age group from birth to age 19. This age group represents 22% of the population (NHS England, 2013), yet accounts for a higher percentage of health service users; for example they make up 26.5% of Accident and Emergency attendances (Health and Social Care Information Centre, 2014). Children and young people have distinct health needs requiring staff that have undergone specialist training in their care in order to meet these needs.

High rates of mental health issues and obesity in English children and young people, plus the worst mortality rates in Europe for 0 to 14-year-old children, are of particular concern to the child health professional (NHS Confederation, 2012), and demand care that promotes good health as well as care for the sick child and young person.

Changes to the way that services for children are configured means there is a need for increased flexibility within the children's nursing workforce. Children's nurses therefore need to be equipped at the point of registration to work across all settings and within integrated children's services teams (Department for Education and Skills, 2004). Fundamentally, children's nurses need to be able to work with a range of different health and social care professionals. See Table 6.2.

Midwife	Hospital play specialist	Nursery nurse
General practitioner	School nurse	Teacher
Health visitor	Social worker	Head teacher
Community paediatrician	Children's nurse (hospital and community)	Dietician
Speech and language therapist	Specialist paediatrician – endocrinology/oncology/orthopaedics	Mental health nurse
Physiotherapist	Education welfare officer	Psychiatrist
Hospital paediatrician	Educational psychologist	Occupational therapist
Learning disability nurse	Voluntary organisations	Chaplain

Table 6.2: Who do children's nurses work with?

Technological advances in neonatal and children's medical care have seen an increase in the number of children surviving into adulthood with ever more complex conditions that require increasing numbers of skilled nurses who are capable of providing the appropriate care in a variety of care settings (the home, hospital, community, respite and palliative care).

The period of adolescence can be challenging for many young people and this requires an in-depth understanding of the physiological changes that are occurring (RCN, 2008). This understanding of adolescence has to be incorporated throughout the various modules of the curriculum, as young people's health and psychological needs are very different from those of a baby or a child. It is important that the newly qualified children's nurse has the necessary knowledge, skills and attributes to deal effectively with their very specific needs.

Lecturer top tip … Ensure that your chosen university and their practice learning opportunities provide the foundations that will equip you with a good grounding in a wide variety of conditions and with children, young people and their families across a variety of settings.

What relevant experience do you have?

It is essential that your personal statement demonstrates that you have experience of working with children and young people and have enjoyed this experience. Think about your work experience, regardless of whether this was as a volunteer or as a paid employee. Have you gained experience of caring for or working with children?

Suggested activities:

- voluntary such as Brownie/Guide/Scout work;
- babysitting;
- child minding;
- nursery nurse;
- work experience in a nursery, children's centre or with a play group;
- healthcare assistant work within a children's ward or children's community care team;
- experience working with children or young people with learning difficulties.

What qualities do children, young people and their families see as important?

The NMC (2010) states that . . .

> *Children's nurses must understand their role as an advocate for children, young people and their families, and work in partnership with them. They must deliver child and family-centred care; empower children and young people to express their views and preferences; and maintain and recognise their rights and best interests.*

Most sick children are cared for in their homes by their close family. However, on occasions, the care required is more specialised and has to be provided by a registered nurse either within the home or at a hospital or hospice. That nurse must be able to work in partnership with the family. The nurse needs to demonstrate certain qualities, such as good communication, trustworthiness, knowledge and safety consciousness, while also maintaining a sense of fun, behaving professionally (by being prompt, respectful and effective) and constantly being aware that the child's family also require care (Brady, 2009; Randall and Hill, 2012).

Nurses need effective communication skills to empower the child, young person and family to deal with the illness and manage the treatment. Often the parents and siblings are in need of care too, as they learn to deal with the psychosocial aspect of seeing the ill child. It is important that the nurse develops an understanding of this and can interpret the family situation and provide holistic care for the child and family. This means that you need excellent listening skills and are able to interpret non-verbal communication. For example, children and young people may not be able to express their feelings about what is happening, but their body language or facial expression may indicate their distress or anger.

Children and young people who have complex care needs often rely on technology such as ventilators, gastrostomy tubes for feeding or a tracheostomy to support their ability to reach their maximum potential. It follows that they and their families expect the nurse to be technologically knowledgeable and able to use a variety of equipment effectively and efficiently (Brady, 2009).

Safeguarding is integral to all aspects of children's nursing. The nurse must be able to use a range of communication techniques such as body language and facial expressions when caring for vulnerable children and young people (NHS Confederation, 2012).

During your practice placements you will meet a wide variety of families that require healthcare, enabling you to gain the knowledge, skills and understanding to be patient and flexible in your approach. It is imperative that you attend to the individual views and opinions of children, young people and their families; since often the nurse is their advocate. Nurses often help the family to make informed decisions that are appropriate to the needs and situation of the child, young person and family, since it is implicit that caring for the whole family is an important aspect of the children's nurse's role.

What qualities do qualified nurses see as important for the children's nurse?

Someone who is able to cope with a high pressured, demanding yet rewarding, varied and interesting, unpredictable job.
Children's community sister

Children's community sister . . . It's not rocket science . . . It's common sense but . . . You need to have good time management . . . be organised, have respect for all people . . . Knowing anatomy and physiology that is related to the patient is important, also being motivated, having the ability to be practical and show initiative . . .

Senior sister, general paediatric ward . . . It's a career . . . you're never too old to start! You could start in your 40s or 50s. Everyone could do it if they had the right personality.

Staff nurse . . . It's very rewarding . . . you come across things that other people wouldn't think happen . . . you're always learning, it never stops . . . There are lots of areas to specialise in . . . It's not a dead end job, you can set yourself goals, there are so many aspects to it, so many things you can do like work on a ward or in the community – what suits one may not suit another . . .

3rd year student nurse [final year] . . . Entering nursing initiates a period of significant personal growth . . . children's nursing nurtures your communication skills to gain a child's trust and voluntary cooperation . . . whether it's by participating in a toddler's fantasy kingdom to unveil their fears and anxieties or identifying with a teen-ager's worshipped music/fashion idol to encourage them to comply with a procedure. Good communication is essential with parents too; from explanations about medical tests and gaining informed consent, breaking bad news and supporting them through difficult phases to discussion about preferred options in care that fit around the child and family . . .

Learning disabilities nursing

Learning disability nursing is probably the least well known of the four fields of nursing. People join the profession for a variety of reasons but they all make a contribution to the care and welfare of a vulnerable group of people (Public Health Division, 2014).

Learning disability nursing is a person-centred profession that supports the wellbeing and social inclusion of people with learning disabilities through improving or maintaining their physical and mental health. We work with service users, their families, and carers across the lifespan.

> Nurse tip . . . Before I saw the advert in the paper I didn't realise that learning disability nursing was a field of nursing that you could study, but if anyone is considering a career in healthcare I would definitely recommend looking into it.

The number of children and adults with learning disabilities is increasing across the United Kingdom and internationally and there has been a steady rise in the number of children and adults with complex needs (Scottish Government, 2012). People who have a learning disability are likely to experience health inequalities; they have higher rates of physical and mental health conditions than their non-disabled peers and experience barriers to accessing effective healthcare (Emerson et al., 2011). It is therefore unsurprising that there is an increasing demand for specialist learning disability services, and learning disability nurses.

Activity 6.2   *What is a learning disability?*

Do you understand what is meant by the term 'learning disability'? Before you write your personal statement it is advisable to undertake some research. As a starting point visit the Foundation for People with Learning Disabilities website at **www.learningdisabilities.org. uk/help-information/about-learning-disabilities/?view=Standard** and explore the information available.

What do learning disabilities nurses do?

Learning disability nursing is a value-based profession, which sees service users as unique with their own specific care needs and places the individual at the centre of planning, devising and delivering their care.

Learning disability nurses work with individuals' families and their carers who have a wide range of strengths and needs, providing evidence-based specialist and generalist nursing care.

Their role has been described as:

- *Maximising health access and outcomes for people through timely evidence-based interventions.*
- *Encouraging and promoting community presence.*

- *Supporting skills teaching and development to maximise independence and good health maintenance.*

- *Providing accurate assessment and implementation of treatment and support to maximise health outcomes.*

- *Using education and health promotion to support carers/families/people to maintain good health.*

- *Supporting non-learning disability specific trained staff in meeting needs of people.*

- *Coordinating care within multi-disciplinary teams to ensure holistic healthcare needs are met.*

- *Challenging and reducing incidence of inequality and discriminatory practice, which affects healthcare outcomes.*

(Thomas, 2014)

How do people with a learning disability see the role of the learning disability nurse?

- They try to understand you and what you want.

- They support us to do the things that are important to us.

- They help to explain why and how you might be treated for health problems.

- They help us to think about ways to keep well and safe.

- They explain how and why you might get treated for health problems.

- They try to find ways to help you that are already proven to work.

- They make sure that you and your supporters(s) know about other people who can help you.

- They know about important new ideas and information that may help you.

- They help us to stop getting unfair treatment.

(Adapted from Department of Health, 2007)

A service user's comment:

> *I'm going into hospital soon and I'm not frightened anymore because (learning disability liaison nurse based in the hospital) will be there to make sure I'm all right.*
> (Scottish Government, 2012)

Where do learning disability nurses work?

Learning disability nursing comprises the largest professional group of qualified staff working within learning disability services (Gates, 2011). They work with children and adults in a wide range of settings and organisations, including the NHS, local authorities and the private, voluntary and statutory sector (Table 6.3). Typically they work in multi-professional teams and in multi-agency settings, such as:

- community learning disability teams;
- specialist community teams/roles, for example working with people who have challenging needs or epilepsy;
- liaison nurse roles supporting access to acute and mental health services;
- inpatient assessment and treatment services for people with additional challenging needs and mental health needs;
- short-break services;
- 24-hour and community-based services for people with profound intellectual and multiple disabilities;
- residential services;
- day services;
- forensic services.

Key skills of a learning disability nurse

We have looked at some of the key attributes and skills required by nurses in Chapter 2, but the following are particularly important for learning disability nurses:

- enhanced communication skills, including non-verbal and alternative communication skills;
- creativity to develop and deliver individualised care plans and resources to address the individual's needs, such as accessible information;
- patience: often work is not about quick fixes and instant results. Relationships and trust can take time to develop: progress is often achieved over long timeframes with many small steps, but the rewards can be great.

General practitioners	Dieticians	Clinical psychologists
School teachers in mainstream and special schools	Speech and language therapists	Drama therapists
School nurses	Adult nurses	Art therapists
Mental health nurses	Children's nurses	Prison services
Social workers	Orthotists	Physiotherapists
Occupational therapists	Music therapists	Psychiatrists

Table 6.3: Who do learning disabilities nurses work with?

Lecturer tip . . . In order to make a good learning disability nurse you need to have an understanding of how it might feel to be a person with a learning disability. One of the best ways to do this is to talk to or hear it from someone who has a learning disability. There are

continued . . .

> many examples you can access online. Here is a link to the MENCAP YouTube site where you can access a number of recordings made by and with people who have a learning disability and their families and see the issues that are important to them: **www.youtube.com/user/ MencapDirector**

What experience is relevant to learning disability nursing?

The experience you are able to gain will depend on your individual situation. If you have friends or family members who have a learning disability then it will be valuable to spend some time getting to know them. Identify their strengths and the challenges they and their family and carers face. It is always helpful to gain an understanding of the client group you hope to work with before you apply. Here are some of the ways you can do this.

- Gain some experience working as a support worker in a residential or day service for people with a learning disability. Bank or agency work can be a good route into this type of work.

- Contact your local special schools for children with severe learning disabilities, asking if they have any volunteer opportunities available.

- Contact your local MENCAP branch (**www.mencap.org.uk**) and ask about volunteer opportunities.

- Contact your local social services department or search online for a list of local organisations providing services to children and adults who have a learning disability. See if any of these services have volunteer opportunities.

A qualified nurse's experience of being a learning disability nurse

> *Nurse view* . . . Becoming a Learning Disability Nurse has changed my life. My practice to date has created an acute awareness of the life challenges and healthcare needs that People with Learning Disabilities face. I want to use my position as a healthcare professional to promote the 'Valuing People Now' agenda . . . If we can get care right for the most vulnerable people in our society this will enable us to get it right for everyone (Daniel Turner, Community Learning Disability Nurse who qualified in 2011).

Mental health nursing

An imbalance in any part of our health can happen at any time, to anyone, and this includes our mental wellbeing. It is widely accepted that one in four of us at some time in our lives will experience a diagnosable mental illness (The Health and Social Care Information Centre, 2009), with one in ten children experiencing mental distress before they reach the age of 16 (The Office for National Statistics, 2005). With an ever-faster lifestyle, an ageing population and increased levels of stressful life events at every corner, the concept of mental distress is predictably increasing. People with mental illness are at a significantly higher risk of experiencing a negative impact on their lifestyle. The rates of serious physical illness, unemployment and overall societal discrimination are significantly higher for those with a mental illness than the general population, with life expectancy for some groups being 25 years shorter than the national average (Royal College of Psychiatrists, 2010). Therefore a professional and highly trained workforce committed to assisting people to recover from their distress, prevent mental health issues occurring and who can combat social exclusion is needed and nursing is a fundamental contributor to this goal.

As a nurse you will need to develop the ability to challenge your own thinking and the views of others in order to attain a wider, more informed view of mental health. Activity 6.3 is a good starting point.

Activity 6.3   *What is your understanding of mental health?*

In order to improve your understanding of mental health, consider for a moment your current thoughts about the subject. Then access the Mind organisation link (**www.mind. org.uk**) to discover a wider viewpoint of the concept and see whether it complements or conflicts with your initial views.

What is mental health nursing?

Just as nursing is hard to define, so is mental health nursing, but the consensus is that it is a profession that places the person at the centre of care and focuses on partnership in order to help people discover new ways of coping and overcoming their illnesses, explore the meaning of their experiences, and discover opportunities for recovery and personal growth beyond just the condition. This occurs within the formation of meaningful and therapeutic relationships (Barker, 2009).

It is clear to see that the emphasis for nurses is to work together with people in partnership whilst holding the person central in the process of recovery. Moving beyond an illness also requires nurses to consider innovative ways in helping people reach their desired quality of life and not merely about removing symptoms. Historically, mental healthcare has been seen largely as a custodial service, a viewpoint still held within some corners of society, which perpetuates a negative view of the purpose of care today. Our challenge as mental health professionals is to combat these outdated views and help service users overcome the unjustified stigma of mental illness.

Nurse view . . . Many people think that mental health nursing is easy; you just sit around all day talking to service users. I'd say that it is the most demanding of all the fields of nursing.

Where do mental health nurses work?

Nurses work in a variety of settings across the age range, from children to older adults in both hospital-based and community care settings. The move towards a greater emphasis on community-based care continues with the goal of treating people in their own homes wherever possible. The overall aim is to maximise a person's independence over their condition and ultimately help people to achieve their future goals in life. In addition, services are wide and varied and are often tailored to the specific needs of individuals through specialist teams. Examples include:

- child and adolescent services and early intervention teams;
- eating disorder services;
- substance misuse services;
- prison and forensic settings;
- crisis and acute care settings;
- rehabilitation and intensive support services;
- older persons' care and dementia services;
- GP and primary care based mental health services.

The diversity in the types of approach available allows mental health nursing to become an exciting and diverse career with the opportunity to experience a wide and rich selection of working environments.

It is important to consider the person and their family or significant others as central to any working partnerships, though Table 6.4 offers some of the different professions you may work with.

General practitioner/general practice teams	Drama therapist mental health support workers
Art therapists: a variety of specialist therapists specialising in family support, music, drama, art and alternative therapies	Counsellors/independent advocates and support staff with lived experience of mental health issues
Occupational therapists	Psychologists
Psychiatrists	Physical healthcare staff including dieticians
Social workers and social care and vocational staff	Clinical nurse specialists, e.g. in eating disorders, substance use and misuse

Table 6.4: Who do mental health nurses work with?

What are the key skills required to work as a mental health nurse?

Service users and their families want nurses to be passionate about the subject and focus on the skill of forming alliances where people are to be listened to and encouraged to be involved in the decisions that affect them. A sense of empowerment and value is important, where all parties are treated as equal within a partnership; these are the foundation blocks if meaningful change is to occur (Gunasekara et al., 2014).

With this in mind the following skills are essential requirements:

- an understanding, empathetic and non-judgmental approach;
- effective communication, listening and interpersonal skills;
- collaborative relationship-building skills;
- a willingness to be innovative and creative in care delivery;
- partnership working with clients, their carers and other health and social care workers to provide a positive experience of care;
- advocacy, negotiation and assertiveness skills;
- the ability to manage challenging situations calmly;
- a broad range of holistic knowledge and practical clinical skills;
- teamwork and leadership skills;
- the ability to relate to and work with people of all ages and from a wide range of cultures;
- the ability to challenge the negative stereotypes and stigma seen in mental health;
- in-depth knowledge and understanding of the most appropriate evidence-based approaches to care.

However, the greatest tool we have as mental health nurses is ourselves. Mental health nurses need to possess unique characteristics, values and attitudes that genuinely demonstrate an interest in engaging with therapeutic relationships with people with mental health issues that lead to a positive experience of care (adapted from Department of Health, 2006; NMC, 2010).

Student nurses' experiences of preparing to become a mental health nurse

Two third-year nursing students (Stefanie Looker and Lucy Riddett) were asked the question: what top tips would you give to people considering a career in mental health nursing? These were a collection of some of their replies:

- *Be assertive, especially on placement to ensure your learning needs are met.*
- *Understand that the course will make you question yourself professionally and personally.*
- *Be organised and prepared for studying and working in practice.*
- *Make sure you get your library books ahead of deadlines and read the reading lists provided.*
- *Ensure you buy a couple of the core text books; ask the lecturers for advice on the most appropriate publications, and consider whether user friendly before purchasing.*

continued . . .

- *Be prepared to balance your social life with work and study commitments.*
- *If you are struggling seek advice as soon as possible, do not leave it and try and face it alone.*
- *Never give up, there is always someone there to talk to in the faculty or other colleagues on the course.*

What experience is relevant to mental health nursing?

To gain experience prior to entering a nursing course, consider paid or voluntary positions that offer a chance to work alongside people with mental health issues. Possible areas are:

- Consider working full/part time in mental health nursing or residential care homes, or day centres;
- NHS and private healthcare assistant roles;
- Explore local and national charities and organisations, such as Mind or Rethink, to discover voluntary opportunities that you can get involved in in your local area.
- Contact social service departments for information on local support groups and buddy schemes you can support.
- Involvement in helplines such as Samaritans and SANE Mental Health Helpline to get links.

Alternatively, spend time speaking to people you may know who have experienced mental distress; find out what was important for them in overcoming their difficulties.

Lecturer tip . . . Visit the Time to Change campaign website (**www.time-to-change. org.uk**). This organisation's goal is to challenge nationally the stigma and discrimination experienced by those with mental health issues. It is a great resource for broadening perspective and knowledge on mental health issues and will help you develop your personal statement.

The future of mental health nursing is at an exciting crossroads, which is at the forefront of minimising the impact of mental illness and preventing future issues from occurring. Nursing intends to strengthen further the working partnerships with service users, families, professional colleagues and within the wider community as a whole, a key concept for future change. The opportunities to become highly skilled and develop as specialists in healthcare are increasing and nursing is seen as a valued body within the field that contributes to care at every level. This includes development in a wide range of holistic skills including medication management and prescribing, psychological therapies, social care coordination and key roles within managerial and educational development. Nurses are at the forefront of a movement to change the perception of mental healthcare, and have a real opportunity not only to work on providing the best treatment available, but also to continue to combat stigma and social exclusion within society wherever it appears.

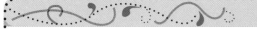

Chapter summary

It is essential that you choose the right field of practice for you. Not all universities offer all four fields of nursing, so having selected your field you will then need to identify which universities offer it. This information is available on the UCAS website and on each university's website. The next chapter will help you to select which of those universities are best suited to your needs.

Further reading

Clarke, V and Walsh, A (2009) *Fundamentals of Mental Health Nursing.* Oxford: Open University Press.

An easy to read text that provides an introductory view into mental health nursing.

Department of Health (2007) *Good Practice in Learning Disability Nursing.* Available from: **http://webarchive.nationalarchives.gov.uk/20130107105354/http://www.dh.gov.uk/en/Publications andstatistics/Publications/PublicationsPolicyAndGuidance/DH_081328**

A useful overview to help you prepare your personal statement and prepare for your selection day.

Hall C et al. (2013) Exploring the world of nursing by those working in it. In Hall, C and Ritchie, D (eds) *What is Nursing? Exploring theory and practice*, 3rd edition. London: Sage/Learning Matters.

This chapter has a series of interviews with nurses from all four fields of nursing which give insight into the field, the skills required and the challenges.

NHS Confederation (2012) *Children and Young People's Health and Wellbeing in Changing Times: Shaping the future and improving outcomes.* Available from: **www.nhsconfed.org/resources/2012/12/children-and-young-peoples-health-and-wellbeing-in-changing-times**

Useful overview that could help you with your personal statement for children's nursing.

Useful websites

www.nhscareers.nhs.uk/nursing.shtml

NHS Careers provides information on all the fields of nursing and the different healthcare professionals they work with.

www.mentalhealth.org.uk

An informative website with an established history of providing information, research and campaigns on the concept mental health within the United Kingdom.

www.ucas.ac.uk

UCAS lists which universities run programmes in each field.

Chapter 7
The application process and choosing the right university

Sue Fergy

Chapter aims

The aim of this chapter is to explore a number of practical considerations to think about before applying to university. By the end of the chapter you will be able to:

- consider what factors might influence your choice of university;
- find out how the universities you are interested in are rated by others;
- understand the process for applying through UCAS;
- identify the key elements that you need to include in your personal statement.

Introduction

Choosing which university to apply to is a big decision and a very personal decision and it is really important to give yourself a lot of time to do the background reading and research to help you make the right decision. Over 60 UK universities offer nursing programmes, so there is a huge choice. There are many ways you can develop a clear picture of what the different universities are offering, for example going to an open day to visit the university campus and accommodation, talking with staff and students, checking out student websites, league tables and the National Student Survey (NSS). There are also a number of 'good university' guides available that are worth reading (both online and in hard copy).

Use this chapter to help you do your research on what is the right university for you. It will be time well spent: remember you will be spending three years of your life there.

Activity 7.1	*What factors are important to me in a university?*

A good place to start is to think about what factors are most important to you, both right now and forecasting what might be important in the coming three to four years. Asking yourself the following questions may help.

1. What field do I want to study and which universities offer it?

Not all universities offer all fields of nursing, for example:

29 universities offer learning disability nursing.

54 universities offer children's nursing.

63 universities offer mental health nursing.

67 universities offer adult nursing.

Not all universities offer the programme you might want, e.g. the postgraduate diploma: only 14 universities offer a postgraduate option.

2. What do I want from my university?

Do I want one at the top of the league tables? Do I want to spend time at a specific hospital trust? Do I need a university with accommodation on site? Do I want a university with good sports facilities? Is it important to me that my university provides excellent support for students with disabilities?

3. Where do I want to live?

Do I want to stay in my current area? Or move closer to friends or family? Do I want to live in a big city or by the coast?

4. If I stay in my current area, what universities are within reasonable travelling distance?

5. How much will it cost to move away? Or to stay at home?

If I move away from home, would I like to live in university or private accommodation? Live with others or live on my own?

6. If I move, how often might I like to visit home?

How much will visiting home cost? Are there good transport links between home and the university?

7. If I want to drive to the university, does the university have parking available for students?

If there is parking, is it free?

Some of these questions may be more important to you than others. It may be useful to identify your priorities and draw up a table to help you compare different universities as you learn more about them. Start with Table 7.1 and adapt it to fit with your important factors.

	Uni. 1	Uni. 2	Uni. 3	Uni. 4	Uni. 5
1. League table position					
2. Cost of university accommodation					
3. Travelling costs to home					
4. Good sports facilities					
5. Free parking available for students					

Table 7.1: Comparison of different universities

The following sections will help you to find out how to answer the questions in Activity 7.1 and complete Table 7.1.

League tables

Each year, a number of university league tables are published. University league tables are lists which compare different aspects of university performance, e.g. entry requirements, teaching quality, staff–student ratio (number of students per member of teaching staff), research activity, career prospects, the proportion of graduates who find graduate-level employment within six months of graduation. League tables are available in book form and online, and are produced by a number of publishers including national newspapers.

A lot of information about universities, including league tables, is published by newspapers in August each year to coincide with the publishing of A level results. League tables are useful sources of information on individual universities and help you to make comparisons, not only between universities in general but how nursing courses compare between different universities. It is a good idea to look at a number of league tables as they all take slightly different approaches to collecting and presenting information. They will be more helpful to you if you have already decided what your priorities are in choosing which university to apply to.

Unistats and the National Student Survey (NSS)

Unistats (**http://unistats.direct.gov.uk**) is the official website to help you make an informed choice when deciding which UK university or college to apply to, based on government statistics. It also includes the results of the latest NSS. The National Student Survey (NSS) is a national survey, which has been conducted by Ipsos MORI annually since 2005. It gathers opinions from final year undergraduates on the quality of their courses. Aimed at current students, the survey asks undergraduates to provide honest feedback on what it has been like to study their course at their institution.

On the Unistats site, you can view a range of university statistics and see how 289,000 students rated their university experience in the latest NSS. You can use Unistats to compare and review universities and subjects in order to help you choose the best UK university and subject for you in light of the following factors: course completion, student achievement, graduate employment, student population (including the percentages of mature, part-time and overseas students) and students' qualifications on entry.

The NSS takes place between February and April each year at most higher and further education institutions across the UK. The NSS gives final-year students an opportunity to give their opinions on what they liked about their time at their university as well as things that could have been better.

The areas that students comment upon are:

- teaching on my course;
- assessment and feedback;
- academic support;
- organisation and management;
- learning resources;
- personal development;
- overall satisfaction.

The information students produce is analysed and presented in an easy-to-use format; universities use this information to develop and improve their programmes.

Travel

When choosing which university to attend, travelling is an issue that requires careful thought. For nursing programmes, there are two elements to travelling. One is how near your university is to the place where you will be living. The second is the travelling involved as part of your pre-registration programme as a student.

A key consideration is where you want to study and how far that is from where your family and friends live. You may want to take this opportunity to go to a university to be nearer to friends in a different part of the country or to live in a city where you have always wanted to live.

If this is the case, think realistically about how often you might want to travel home, how flexible the transport routes are and how much the journey would cost. If most of your friends and family live in the north of England, studying in London would mean long and perhaps expensive journeys to visit them, which means you might not be able to do that often.

A second consideration is the travelling involved while on the programme. If you decide to apply to a university quite close to where you currently live (so that you do not have to move), you still need to think about how easy it will be to travel to the university for a 9 o'clock start, which is often the start time for university lectures (and punctuality is really important for nurses). A short journey from one part of a large city to another might involve two or three changes of transport, including buses and trains; long journeys could mean getting up very early several mornings in a row – fine in June but more of a challenge in January. How good are the transport links? Is there a university bus you could use? If you drive, is there on-site parking available for students? Is it free? Following a consideration of all of these factors, you might decide you want to live in university accommodation; therefore you need to check out what this is like at the universities you are interested in and how much it costs. Also find out if it is available for the first year only, or your whole programme.

The next thing to think about is travelling to and from practice placements from where you live. You will be spending 50% of your course in practice: in hospitals, clinics, residential homes, GP surgeries or visiting patients' homes. It is really important to find out where your favourite universities allocate their students to gain their practice experience. Many university websites will tell you about the healthcare settings they use for student practice experiences.

In lots of care settings, nurses undertake shift work and it is a requirement of the Nursing and Midwifery Council that student nurses have experience of caring for patients throughout a range of shift patterns so that you have an understanding of the patient's journey throughout 24 hours of care. This means you **will** be doing shift work – including night duty!

> Lecturer tip . . . Travelling time to some of your placements may take up to two hours each way, so check what a university may expect to be reasonable travel times and consider how you would manage this.

Go back to Activity 2.3 in Chapter 2 and complete it for the universities you are interested in. This will give you an idea of both travel times and costs and whether you can realistically manage these for the universities you have chosen.

> Student tip . . . Before I started at the university, I experimented a bit with the local transport to find out which ways were quickest and which ways were cheapest. For a 9 a.m. start I choose the quickest way, but when we start later, I choose the cheapest route.

Disability support

We discussed in Chapter 2 the issue of applying for a nursing course if you have a disability so, if this is of relevance to you, refer back there to refresh your mind.

Each university publishes a disability statement explaining how it provides support to students with disabilities. As a potential student, you can ask to see a copy of this statement, or look for it on the university's website.

If you have a disability, you may find it useful to contact a university's disability adviser or learning support co-ordinator before you make a final decision about where to study. If you don't find them very helpful, then maybe that university isn't the right one for you.

Open days and higher education events

Universities hold open days throughout the year where you can visit the university campus and meet with academic staff who will be teaching the courses you are interested in and students who are already on the course. UCAS also runs around 50 conventions a year where you can meet representatives from universities and discuss the courses they offer and the options available. Attending these days and events can help you to finalise your decision as to which universities seem right for you. Details of open days can be found on university websites and the UCAS events website (**www.ucas.com/news-events/events**).

UCAS application process

Once you have chosen your preferred course of study and your preferred universities, you can then apply; for nursing you can apply for up to five different courses. A word of advice here: it is usually a mistake to apply for courses in two different fields of nursing at the same university. It shows a lack of certainty – or that you have not done enough research and you are unlikely to get very far with that application.

The UCAS website offers very detailed help and advice to guide you throughout the entire process including a section called 'How it all works' (**www.ucas.com/how-it-all-works**). One of the first things you will need to get started is an e-mail address, as this is how UCAS and the university will communicate with you, so if you don't have one already, sign up for one now. E-mail accounts can be set up for free via the internet: the most popular are Gmail (run by Google), Windows Live Hotmail (owned by Microsoft), AOL and Yahoo! Mail. Even if you already have an email account for social use, you might want to open a new one for career purposes e.g. Jess.Smith1992@gmail.com has a different feel to QT.Hotlips@hotmail.com!

When applying for university admission, you will need to complete an online UCAS form. Read through each section to get a feel of what information is required so that when you sit down to complete your application form you have everything you need in front of you. The information that will be required is:

- your personal details;
- additional information on ethnic origin and national identity, activities in preparation for higher education, care and parental education and occupational background;
- the universities you wish to apply to;
- your previous educational achievements;
- details of any previous employment you have had;
- your personal statement.

There are different deadlines for different subjects and so it is crucial that you apply before the deadline set for your particular course. If you miss the deadline, you might well miss starting university in the year you were hoping to start. Generally the deadline is mid-January for nursing courses that start in September, but check the UCAS website for details as some universities offer programmes starting at other times of the year and many offer places through clearing in August (see Chapter 12).

Writing your personal statement

An important part of the application process is writing your personal statement. It is important because this is your very first, personal and official contact with the university. Your application is your first foot in the door and if the personal statement lets you down, that's as far as this application is going. Because it is so important, it is worth giving it a lot of time to plan and perfect, seeking advice and asking for help from people who are on your side (friends and family) and from the experts (teachers, lecturers, university admissions staff).

Lecturer tip . . . As an admissions tutor, I read hundreds of personal statements a year. If a personal statement has spelling or grammatical errors in it, it immediately raises questions for me about the candidate. For a start – can the person spell? Is the applicant able to write grammatically correct sentences? Or is this applicant just careless? Either way, it makes me think they are not particularly committed to or suitable for my nursing programme. There will be hundreds of personal statements that are very much better.

Your personal statement will need to stick to the very detailed and strict guidelines laid down by UCAS. These include:

Using 4000 characters, including lines and spaces. Using no more than 47 lines.

One suggestion is to work on your personal statement as a Word document before copying it into your application form. Word (and other similar programmes) can give you a character count so you know exactly how many you have used. What needs to be clear in your personal statement is your understanding and enthusiasm for the course you are applying for and why you are the right person for it.

The personal statement is an opportunity for you to demonstrate your understanding of what nursing requires. If you have qualities such as maturity and a high level of personal commitment, open-mindedness, patience and determination, then your statement should highlight how you feel you can demonstrate these qualities through real examples in your life. Illustrate how you would cope with the challenges and demands that a career in nursing could present you with, and give examples of how you have managed such challenges before.

You should also have demonstrable practical experience, and the personal statement is the best place to outline this. If you do not have work experience in healthcare, then you should look at work experience you have had and relate the skills and experiences you have gained to nursing.

See Chapter 4 on work experience. You should also have awareness of current healthcare affairs: healthcare issues frequently hit television and newspaper headlines, and if you are up to date with current issues, university admissions tutors can see your commitment to the course of study.

It is really important that you are scrupulously honest in your personal statement. Make sure that you would be happy to answer questions on any of the points you have made. You need to ensure that the statement is a true reflection of your life and includes the reasons why you have decided to do nursing. Your statement needs to stand out from the others and be memorable, and the best way to do that is to give real-life examples that you would be able to talk about at the interview if you were asked. It is also crucial that it is you who writes your personal statement; do not be tempted to download one from the Internet or copy from a friend. UCAS runs a similarity detection service to ensure that personal statements are written by the individual applicant who is making the application.

The very helpful UCAS website offers some tools to make this process easier – including a video on dos and don'ts – on a webpage called 'Your personal statement': **www.ucas.com/how-it-all-works/undergraduate/filling-your-application/your-personal-statement**

Activity 7.2 will get you started.

Activity 7.2 — *What to put in your personal statement*

Look at Table 7.2 and make some short sentences in the third column. You can then use these to start developing your personal statement.

Get other people who you know and trust to read your statement and comment on it; ask them to be critical. These people may be your teachers, careers advisers, tutors at college or parents.

The UCAS website includes a useful section on why applications were not successful and shares the following comments specifically about personal statements.

Your personal statement does not strongly support your desire to study your chosen degree.

*Your personal statement did not show sufficient understanding, relevance or knowledge about the course you are applying for. (UCAS website, **www.ucas.ac.uk**, 2011)*

UCAS (2011) noted that the phrase 'Nursing is a very challenging and demanding career' was used in 275 personal statements, so ensure your statement shows some originality.

On a serious note, UCAS operates a dedicated Verification Team whose job it is to prevent and detect fraud and similarity in personal statements. UCAS explains its aim:

Our aim is to avoid anyone gaining from an unfair advantage and securing a place by deception. If you provide true, complete and accurate information and if your personal statement is all your own work, then you have nothing to worry about.

So, it's important to keep it honest and personal. The Which University website offers advice from admissions tutors (**http://university.which.co.uk/advice/personal-statements-the-student-guide-to-selling-yourself**).

UCAS personal statement	Some examples	Your example
How you have researched the nursing profession	Speaking to practising nurses, reading the nursing press, watching health-related TV programmes	
How you have worked with vulnerable people or worked within teams where you may have developed skills that may be relevant to nursing	Volunteering in a charity shop, co-ordinating the rota at the youth club or helping organise a jumble sale	
How you have gained insight into the course	Going to open days, UCAS events, talking to students already on the course	
Why you have chosen your specific field of nursing and what the challenges of that field are	Relate to work or personal experiences. To find out more about each field, see Chapter 6	
Your personal qualities that relate to nursing	If you are compassionate, give an example of where you have helped a friend in need or cared for someone at work. Refer back to Chapter 2	
Hobbies and interests	Need to relate to skills/qualities needed in nursing in some way. For example, you like team games (team player); you enjoy volunteering at the football club (organisational skills)	

Table 7.2: UCAS personal statement

Further sources of help and advice for potential students

There are a number of websites dedicated to offering support and advice to potential students and it is a growing area. So, in the search engine of your choice, search for 'top student websites' or 'best student websites' to find out whether any new sites have popped up recently. Below are some of the most useful ones we have found, which can provide information ranging from how to choose a university, to students' own experiences of attending selection days and students' views on what is great and not so great at their university. Each of these sites can help you to shortlist your final university choices.

UCAS

UCAS is the organisation responsible for managing applications to higher education courses in the UK and would be your first port of call. UCAS processes applications for full-time undergraduate programmes – nearly two million every year. It has sections for students, parents, people who advise potential students and a section for university staff to help keep up to date with application processes.

The UCAS site (**www.ucas.com**) is very user-friendly, offering a number of short videos giving advice on all aspects of the application process. It also hosts a number of discussion boards and forums for people who are in the process of applying to university; this gives you the opportunity to ask questions of people who are in the same boat as you and share your experiences and opinions. It also offers advice on writing personal statements, advice on UK tariffs and, most importantly, advice on application deadlines; if you miss a deadline your application may well not be processed.

Once you have submitted your application, UCAS is also the place where you can check whether you have been made an offer.

UCAS also has a section for people who already have degrees, UKPASS (**www.ukpass.ac.uk**), which is an online postgraduate application service.

The Student Room

The Student Room is the UK's largest student website (**www.thestudentroom.co.uk**) and contains a wide range of essential student resources, including the world's busiest student forum. All the content is written by students for students. The Student Room has over 1.5 million members. The site also contains tens of thousands of university reviews, personal statements, revision notes and articles written by a range of students. The Student Room is the biggest academic and social student resource in the UK.

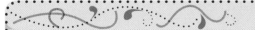

Chapter summary

This chapter has identified some of the factors you need to consider when choosing which universities to apply to and offered you a range of resources that will provide you with further information to help you shortlist them to the final five. Once you have your shortlist, the UCAS website will take you step by step through the application process and keep you informed about the progress of your applications. Take plenty of time preparing your personal statement; this is what will make you stand out from other applicants and gain you an interview. Once you have secured that all-important interview date you need to consider how you will prepare for it, which is what we will look at in the next chapter.

Further reading

Borrego, M and Baird, J (2010) *Careers Uncovered: Nursing and midwifery*, 2nd edition. Richmond: Trotman.

This book gives a useful overview of careers in nursing and midwifery. It provides information about applying for nursing and offers detailed insights into the four fields of nursing. It also advises you on how to apply for your first job as a registered nurse. It contains a number of case studies of real nurses, tracing their professional progress from the beginning of their careers to their current positions.

Tobin, L (2009) *A Guide to Uni Life: The one stop guide to what university is REALLY like.* Richmond: Trotman.

Written by a student this book provides guidance on surviving at university from freshers' week through to the end of your course.

The UCAS Guide to Getting into University and College: Everything you need to know about the entire research and application process (2012), 2nd revised edition, UCAS.

This book advertises itself as 'everything you need to know about the entire application and research process'. It could be a very useful text for students who are not in school or college and might therefore not be able to receive advice from experienced teachers on the UCAS process.

Useful websites

NHS bursaries

For updated information on bursaries and other financial support go to:

England: **www.nhsbsa.nhs.uk/Students.aspx**

Northern Ireland: **http://www.nidirect.gov.uk/nhs-and-social-work-students**

Scotland: **www.saas.gov.uk/full_time/nmsb/index.htm**

Wales: **www.wales.nhs.uk/sitesplus/955/page/72050**

For the bursary estimate calculator

www.ppa.org.uk/StudentBursariesCalculator/reset.do

Additional websites

http://nursing.nhscareers.nhs.uk/skills/what_skills

NHS Careers provides some useful guidelines on the type of skills needed in nursing that can help you write your personal statement.

www.nmc-uk.org/Approved-Programmes

The Nursing and Midwifery Council website has a database in which you can search all the higher education institutes which run pre-registration nursing programmes.

www.nus.org.uk

The National Union of Students (NUS) has a helpful website section, entitled Advice, where you can find tips and hints and information on becoming a student, settling in at university, money and funding issues, study tips and advice on housing issues.

www.thecompleteuniversityguide.co.uk

This site offers detailed information on how to apply to university; it also has profiles of all UK universities.

National Student Survey website: **www.thestudentsurvey.com**

Unistats: **https://unistats.direct.gov.uk**

Chapter 8
Preparing for the selection day

Kim Tolley

> **Chapter aims**
>
> The aim of this chapter is to explore how you prepare for your nursing selection day. By the end of the chapter you will be able to:
>
> - recognise the areas that you need to prepare for the selection day;
> - list the items that you need to take with you;
> - find information that will help you prepare for the selection day;
> - consider how you will present yourself.

Introduction

> Student view . . . I looked at the letter and knew that it was about my nursing application. I recognised the university stamp on the envelope. I have an interview in three weeks' time! Then the reality sank in. I really want to get on this course and if I am successful it will be the start of my career in a job that I really want to do. I knew that I really needed to be well prepared to make sure I had the best chance of getting in.

You have crossed the first major bridge in applying successfully and getting an interview; this is the first step on your journey. Your application form has been vetted by the university admissions tutor who has shortlisted you to come for a selection event. This in itself is a real achievement; this selection event is your opportunity to show your interviewers what you are really like as a person and why you are well suited to being a nurse. You need to be well prepared for this day so that you transform your application into a place on the course.

So far all the university has seen of you is your application and personal statement, but gaining a place on a nursing course requires much more than the ability to express yourself on paper. At the selection day they will want to ensure that you have the necessary skills, knowledge and attitudes required to complete the nursing programme and become a qualified nurse. Completing the programme once you are selected is crucial to both you and the university as they aim to reduce drop-out rates, which cost them money and you disappointment. So it is essential that you are well prepared for this day and take some time to think about the key issues. If you follow this chapter and undertake all the activities and suggestions this will give you the best possible chance of success on the day.

In Chapter 2 we looked at the type of work that nurses do; it is vital that you have a clear understanding of this for the selection day. Other areas in which this chapter will help prepare you for the selection day are:

- planning for the day;
- the journey;
- how you present yourself;
- how to prepare yourself for the format of the day;
- what to take with you;
- what reading you can do;
- dos and don'ts.

Interview preparation

It is strongly recommended that you read nursing journals and articles about healthcare before your interview. Some knowledge of current affairs within nursing will help you feel prepared for any questions and show that you have thought carefully about your career choice. The BBC health website (**www.bbc.co.uk/news/health**) is also a good resource for topical news stories.

Activity 8.1   *Getting inside information*

Take a look at the website the Student Room (**www.thestudentroom.co.uk**). You can post questions on here, but also search for information about the universities and the courses you have applied for. Very often students share their experiences of interview formats. While universities do regularly change their questions it may give you a better feel for what to expect. Note the type of questions asked and think about how you might answer them.

It is not a good idea to write out and rote-learn full answers to possible questions you may be asked at your selection day. First, it shows, and sounds false; second, the question asked may be slightly different from what you expect and will either throw you completely or you'll give your rote answer, which will be wrong, and lastly many universities don't use a traditional interview format anymore as the focus is on selecting people with the right values (called values-based recruitment) so check out the university website to find out what approach they use for selecting students and see Chapter 11 for more guidance on the different selection methods now being used. However, to start you thinking about key areas which may be covered, write out key points in answer to these questions:

- What is the role of a nurse?

- What does a nurse actually do?

- Why have you chosen nursing as a career?

- Why have you chosen this particular programme of study? The different ways of qualifying as a nurse are reviewed in Chapter 3.

- Why have you chosen the adult/child/learning disability/mental health field?

- Where do you see yourself in five years?

- What are your strengths?

- What are your weaknesses?

- How do you manage stress?

- Give an example of where you have been part of a team.

- Summarise any work experience that you have had (and see Chapter 4).

- How will you manage studying whilst on placements?

- Have you considered the impact of the course on your lifestyle?

Ask someone you trust to give you a mock interview. If you can, choose someone who has experience in healthcare or human resources. Discuss with this person what you are going to wear and practise entering a room, smiling, maintaining eye contact and shaking hands. These are essential skills for setting the tone of the interview and it is vital that you get this right to make a good first impression.

Student tip . . . Have a look on YouTube for some interview tips and examples; these are fun to watch and good preparation.

Preparing for numeracy and literacy tests

Most universities now test the numeracy and literacy skills of their applicants to nursing. If any of your chosen universities test for these they may send examples; otherwise check their website for sample tests. If you have any difficulties with the tests, read Chapters 9 and 10, which also have recommended websites and books to help you further.

Criminal records

We discussed in Chapter 3 the importance of declaring on your UCAS application form any criminal convictions, warnings or reprimands you may have had. In Chapter 3 we considered the system for checking and monitoring of previous criminal convictions and cautions, etc. which changed in 2013 to a new system known as the Disclosure and Barring Service. If you have had contact with the police the admissions team may wish to discuss this with you at your selection day and it will be helpful to take any information you have with you. For example:

- date of conviction;
- type of conviction (e.g. conviction, warning, reprimand, fine);
- explanation of the event that led to the conviction;
- whether your circumstances have changed since the conviction;
- what you have learnt from the experience – this is the most important part and is what the interviewers will want to discuss with you if they need to bring this up.

Planning for the day

Book the day off from your current job or tell your college or school that you have an interview. Many selection days last a whole day. If you need reasonable adjustments because of a disability on the selection day, such as extra time for the literacy test or hard copies of the presentations, then make sure that you tell the university well beforehand. If you are not sure who to talk to, contact the disability team at the university and they will advise you. You will be asked to show them your needs assessment if you have dyslexia. We have already explained in Chapter 2 that this will not prevent you from entering nursing, but if the university is aware that you have a disability then they can ensure that you are not disadvantaged in any way on the selection day and are able to show them your best abilities.

Before you completed your application form you will have read up about the university and looked at ratings such as their National Student Survey scores and its place in the university league tables. Remind yourself of these again before the interview and jot down any questions you may have. It is important that the university feels you have made an informed choice to apply there specifically and having this knowledge will help.

> Lecturer tip … Remember, it's not just about the university choosing you, but you choosing it as well.

The journey to the selection day

It is important to start with the practicalities of the selection event. This may seem obvious, but if you organise these things first this will help you to feel ready to do your best on the day and will start to relieve some of your anxieties. So first, how are you going to get there? You may have been to the university before, perhaps on an open day, but this would have been on a different day of the week, perhaps at a weekend and parking and public transport may be very different on your selection day.

Getting to any interview on time is most important. Again it might seem obvious, but a delayed journey can have a huge impact on your ability to do your best on the day. Arriving early will give you the opportunity to have a coffee and calmly get ready for the interview. It is also a good opportunity to soak up the atmosphere of the university, have a look round and observe how the students interact with each other.

Planning the journey is the first step and is a skill that you will use when you are on the programme and have to go out on placements to areas where you may not have been before. If you are late, this shows the interviewers that you may not be able to cope with these challenges. So preparation is the key.

Activity 8.2   *Planning your journey*

Go on the university website and locate the building where your interview will be. Print off a plan of the campus to take with you on the day and mark on it where you have to go.

Consider your journey: are you travelling by car or public transport? You may be coming from a long way away, or you may live a few miles from the campus. Wherever you are travelling from, the same principles apply. If at all possible you need to do a 'dummy run' of the journey in advance of the big day.

Student view . . . I live about ten miles from the university and had driven past it many times. My aunt had driven me to the open day a few months ago so I knew where to park. I decided to practise one morning at about the same time I had to get there for my selection day. The traffic was much worse than I had expected and I realised that I would have to allow an extra 30 minutes for the journey. When I arrived at the campus I found the car park, but realised that I would have to allow time to go to reception to get a parking permit for the day and this also added 15 minutes to my journey. Thank goodness I had tried this out before the actual day, when I knew that I would be panicking anyway!

Creating the right image

Remember the interviewing staff will be assessing you from the moment you arrive. When you check in with the staff it is important to smile and to have all your paperwork to hand. If there is a talk before the interview it is important to look interested and engaged. If you feel able, ask a relevant question, but don't feel that you have to, as all your questions may have been covered.

Lecturer tip . . . First impressions really do count. This is particularly important in nursing, as when we meet other nurses, patients, service users or members of the multidisciplinary team it is vital to be approachable and polite. Patients make instant judgments about how professional nurses are, so bear this in mind and apply the same principles to your interview.

What you wear is also an important part of creating the right impression. The golden rule is be comfortable, but smart. Try out what you are going to wear and ask your friends to be critical. Although it is controversial we have to recognise that judgments are made the instant someone meets you, so don't wear jeans or trainers as they are too casual for an interview. It may seem obvious, but make sure your interview clothes are clean and well ironed. Think carefully about issues such as make-up; do not wear too much. Think also about piercings. These are not allowed in nursing practice; only a single stud earring is allowed in most placement areas, so it may be best not to have them in at interview. When you are nursing you also have to think about smell. Do you smell of cigarette smoke or strong perfume or after-shave? Again think about how you would expect a nurse to present themselves professionally and see if you can mirror this.

> Lecturer tip . . . Attention to detail is very important and if it seems you have not paid attention to your appearance your commitment may be questioned.

What to take with you

In the letter inviting you for interview there will be specific instructions about what time to arrive for the interview and what to bring with you. You will be asked to bring specific documents, such as your passport, and proof of address such as a utility bill. These may be used to complete the disclosure and barring forms. Table 8.1 is a checklist to help you ensure that you

	Tick
The letter inviting you for the interview	
Directions	
A copy of your UCAS application form (it is good to have read this before you attend, to remind yourself what you have written on your personal statement)	
A notebook and pen, to write down notes from the presentation	
Your portfolio	
Certificates that you have been asked to bring, for example from your Access course, BTEC, GCSEs, A levels, Highers etc.	
Identification that you have been asked to bring, for example: • passport; • marriage certificate; • birth certificate; • utility bill.	
A list of any questions you need to have answered. For example, do you understand what type of assessments you will have during the course, how far you would need to travel, whether you would be going to one geographical area for your placements or if these are spread out?	

Table 8.1: What to take with you to the interview

remember to take everything with you. It is useful to keep all these documents in a wallet ready for each interview, and then you won't be searching for them on the day. This demonstrates that you are organised when you arrive and are asked for your papers. You may wish to add to the list in Table 8.1 as you are invited to other interviews, as different universities may ask for different items.

Final dos and don'ts

Do:

- prepare everything the night before;
- smile;
- let the admissions team know in advance of the day if you require any reasonable adjustments;
- take the documents that they have asked for;
- look smart;
- wear layers so if you get hot you can remove some layers;
- look around the university setting: does it suit you, would you fit in there?
- listen to other students in the canteen or coffee shop: what are they saying about the university?
- think about clinical placements: how easy would it be for you to get there at 7 a.m. or get home in the evening?
- ask if they offer a tour at the interview if you have not been able to go on an open day tour;
- jot down after the interview the positive and negative things about the interview and university; this will help you chose which one is best for you.

Don't:

- wear uncomfortable clothing;
- rote-learn answers – it shows;
- make any judgments until you have been to the interview.

> *Student view* ... I arrived early and sat in the university coffee shop in the entrance to the library. There was a real mix of students, across all age groups and cultures. Students were chatting to their friends and some were working on the internet, looking at their e-mails. The place had a real buzz about it and I could see myself fitting in there.

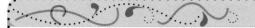

Chapter summary

This chapter has considered how you can prepare for your selection day. The better prepared you are, the more confident you will feel. Information is power and so the more information you can get about the universities where you have interviews and the more reading around you have done about what nursing is and the career options available, the more in control you will feel on the big day. Chapters 9 and 10 will help prepare you for the specifics of the numeracy and literacy elements and Chapter 11 will discuss the key elements of the selection day in more detail and help you further in your preparations.

Useful websites

www.bbc.co.uk/news/health

The BBC health website is a good resource for topical news stories which you could be asked about.

http://nursing.nhscareers.nhs.uk

A website about nursing careers, aimed at people interested in becoming a nurse.

http://www.ucas.com/ucas/conservatoires/apply-and-track/auditions-and-offers/interview-tips

UCAS provides excellent advice on how to prepare for your interview.

Chapter 9
Numeracy tests

Andrew Perkins

Chapter aims

This chapter looks at the different types of calculation you are likely to see in numeracy tests set by universities as part of their selection criteria. By the end of this chapter, you will:

- appreciate why numeracy is an important skill for nurses;
- understand which numeracy skills are important;
- be able to identify areas where you need to improve;
- be familiar with the types of questions you will be asked at selection days.

Introduction

Most universities providing nurse education programmes require you to sit a numeracy test as part of their selection procedure, even if you have A-level maths. This usually happens on your interview day and is likely to cover basic maths skills such as calculations involving decimals, fractions, percentages and metric conversions. In this chapter we will explain why numeracy is so important and give examples of the types of question you may see on your selection days (and some techniques to solve them).

Are you a maths person, or not?

If the word 'numeracy', especially when combined with 'test', sends a shudder down your spine, then this chapter is for you. If you are good with figures, try the practice tests in Activities 9.1–9.10 to check you are up to speed. Never forget there is a very important connection between numeracy and nursing, which allows you to administer safe care for your patients. There is more on this later in the chapter.

For many of us there is a certain mystique concerning numbers which can quickly develop into fear. Almost daily, when challenged with a numerical problem, this fear is often covered up with expressions such as 'I don't do maths'. It is easy to draw a sort of comfort and protection from this, especially if others around you agree that they 'don't do maths' either. Unfortunately in nursing you will have to do maths. It cannot be avoided; but don't worry, this chapter will help you!

Why is numeracy important?

If you said two tablets – well done! If you gave a different answer you may have either given your patient an overdose or not have given him enough. Either scenario could have a serious impact on his recovery. However, numeracy is not just about drug calculations. Numeracy skills are also required to enable you to undertake a range of tasks, such as measuring body mass index which is important when looking at a person's nutritional status. You will use numeracy skills for adding up and balancing fluid input and output charts which enable a patient's fluid balance to be monitored to ensure that they are not dehydrated or given too much fluid. Each of these skills will be taught during your programme, but you do need an understanding of maths to apply these skills safely and effectively.

Calculators

First, a word about calculators. Calculators are a quick and (usually) accurate way of dealing with both simple and more complicated calculations. Just like computers, however, the information given out is only as good as the information put in. If you hit a wrong number by mistake, the answer will inevitably be wrong. This is also true for calculations involving decimal figures. If you put the decimal point in the wrong place, it will be in the wrong place in the answer. You also need to know what sum to do in the first place. Calculators should, therefore, be used with caution. Always estimate in advance what a sensible answer would be and compare this with what the calculator displays, before noting it down. There is more on this later (see sections on decimal calculations and multiplying fractions, below). In summary, you cannot rely on a calculator to do your maths thinking for you. In nursing, you need to understand what you are doing with figures and be able to check each and every calculation you make for accuracy. Having said all this, it is unlikely that you will be allowed to use a calculator in your numeracy test at your interview day.

The numeracy test

What of the test itself? How difficult is it going to be? Generally, numeracy tests are set at GCSE level (level 2). Unlike GCSE, where you can pass with 40% accuracy, in the profession of nursing you always need to be 100% accurate. In fact the Nursing and Midwifery Council (NMC) requires you to achieve 100% in numeracy by the end of graduate training and you will find that when you apply for your first job after qualifying that you will be asked to attend an assessment centre where they will expect you to achieve 100% again. However, the interview test will not ask you to be that much of a genius! The assessors just want you to show that you have a good grasp of the basic numeracy skills you will need to calculate amounts of fluid or the correct dose of a drug that can be administered safely to a patient. Don't worry, though. During your course, you will find there are ready-made, easy-to-follow formulae that help you arrive at the right answer. First, though, you must demonstrate that you know the basics and that's what the numeracy test at the selection day is all about. Again, you can go directly to the practice tests now if you like and see how you get on or have a quick look and come back here.

The test is likely to include straightforward adding up, taking away, multiplying and dividing questions and metric conversions. Some of these will contain numbers with decimal points and others, calculations involving fractions, percentages and ratios. There may also be questions related directly to healthcare such as finding the percentage weight loss of a patient or a dose to be given in accordance with their weight. So, make sure you obtain specimen tests on which to practise, to avoid surprises.

Maths terms

- number: the way we describe an amount, e.g. four biscuits, six years old, 3.24 km, size 38 shoes, £53;

- numeral: a number written in figures, rather than words, e.g. 4, 56, 7.32;

- digit: one numeral in a number, e.g. 3560 has four digits: 3, 5, 6 and 0;

- mixed number: one that includes a whole number and parts or fractions of a whole. Mixed numbers can be expressed as decimals (with a point dividing the whole and the parts) or fractions.

Decimal calculations

If you're already thinking, 'I never know where the decimal point goes in the answer', then you just need to follow some basic rules. These will be helpful when you come to calculating safe doses for your patients. When you are setting out the question for adding, taking away and division, keep the decimal point in line. For example:

Adding

| 2.3 + 5.2 | or | 35.08 + 27.1 |

$$
\begin{array}{r}
2.3 \\
+ 5.2 \\
\hline
= 7.5
\end{array}
\qquad
\begin{array}{r}
35.08 \\
+ 27.1 \\
\hline
= 62.18
\end{array}
$$

You have to do the same for taking away (subtracting).

Subtracting

For example:

9.5 − 2.3   or   85.2 − 61.29

$$\begin{array}{r} 9|.|5 \\ -\,2|.|3 \\ \hline = 7|.|2 \end{array} \qquad \begin{array}{r} 85|.|2 \\ -\,61|.|29 \\ \hline = 23|.|91 \end{array}$$

You also have to do the same for dividing.

Dividing

For example:

260.8 ÷ 4

$$4\,\overline{|260\,|.|8}\;\;{}^{65\,|.|2}$$

5629.82 ÷ 7

$$7\,\overline{|5629\,|.|82}\;\;{}^{804\,|.|26}$$

The same applies for long division. For example:

6412.12 ÷ 13

$$\begin{array}{r} 493|.|24 \\ 13\,\overline{|6412|.|12} \\ 52 \\ \hline 121 \\ 117 \\ \hline 42 \\ 39 \\ \hline 31 \\ 26 \\ \hline 52 \\ 52 \\ \hline 00 \end{array}$$

Answer: 493.24

Note that there are two digits after the decimal point. This is known as 'two decimal places'.

Just before we leave division with decimals, you may find that you are asked to divide using a decimal figure. You simply move the decimal point to the right and do the same with the figure you are dividing into. For example:

24 ÷ 2.5 (or 2.5 into 24) becomes 2. 5 = 25

and 24 (really it's 24.0) becomes 24. 0 = 240

You then continue with long division (240 ÷ 24) as usual. (The answer is 9.6.)

For decimal numbers divided by decimal numbers, it's the same thing. For example:

273.6 ÷ 0.8 (0.8 into 273.6) becomes 0. ↷ 8 = 8

and 273.6 becomes 273. ↷ 6 = 2736

(The answer is 342.)

Multiplying

For smaller numbers and some larger ones it is a good idea to estimate what the answer might be. This will help when you come to doing healthcare calculations because if the answer seems unreasonable then it very probably is. Put another way, if the medicine won't fit in a medicine pot, you are likely to have made a mistake in the calculation.

For example, by using only the whole numbers from the calculation 3.1×2.2 (that is, 3 and 2), multiplying them would give you 6, so the answer must be roughly 6:

$$3.1 \times 2.2$$
$$\downarrow \quad \downarrow$$
$$3 \times 2 = 6 \text{ (and a little bit more)}$$

At least, then, you will know that your answer will be between 6 and 7, and cannot be 60, 600 or 6,000 and something.

The other thing you will see is that there is a digit after the decimal point after the '3' and another after the '2'. This makes two decimal figures in all:

$$3 . 1 \times 2 . 2$$

You can use this information to put the decimal point in the right place when you have finished the calculation. You start by multiplying in the usual way but ignoring the decimal points, for now:

```
    31
 ×  22
   620
 +  62
   682
```

The answer is 682 but, remembering that there were originally two digits after the decimal points, you now count back two places from the right:

6. 8 2   So the point goes here at 6 (and a little bit more)

Try the practice questions in Activity 9.1.

Activity 9.1   *Adding, taking away, multiplying and dividing decimals*

1. $13.7 + 5.8$ =
2. $57.2 + 6.08$ =
3. $0.19 + 1.96$ =
4. $15.72 - 11.01$ =
5. $43.96 - 13.97$ =
6. $34.3 - 24.03$ =

7. 2.2×3.9 =
8. 24.9×11.2 =
9. 53.08×8.5 =
10. $19.6 \div 8$ =
11. $77.6 \div 1.6$ =
12. $826.65 \div 3.3$ =

The answers to Activity 9.1 are given at the end of the chapter.

Fractions to decimals and back to fractions

The next set of questions (Activity 9.2) refers to the conversion of fractions to decimals.

Have a look at Figure 9.1. The chart concerns place value, which means that the value of a digit depends on its place in a number.

On the far left is a column for the 1000s and to the right of that, one column each for the hundreds, tens and units. It's the placing of the figures (including the nought) in the correct column which tells you whether you have a large figure, such as 2074, or a smaller one, 274.

Look at the '1' in the units column. When measuring something it doesn't always come to an even number. The '1', therefore, has to be split into smaller pieces. This gives rise to the tenths (1/10ths) column to the right of the units. The '1' is split into 10 pieces: one-tenth, two-tenths, three-tenths, and so on, up to nine-tenths. As fractions, these are written 1/10, 2/10, up to 9/10. Add another 1/10 and you are back to the total of 1 again.

The other thing to note on the chart is that there are decimal points between the units column and the 10ths column. This means that 0.3, for example, is the same as 3/10 and 0.7 is the same as 7/10. You can prove it, too, by dividing the 10 into the 3 and the 10 into the 7:

$$10\overline{)3.^30} \quad = 0.3 \qquad \text{and} \qquad 10\overline{)7.^70} \quad = 0.7$$

So, for every fraction that is a 1/10th (has a 10 underneath), there is nothing to calculate to find the decimal equivalent. It's the same thing. For fractions that don't have a 10 underneath, you will have to divide the bottom into the top, as above. For example, 1/8 as a decimal would be worked out like this:

$$8\overline{)1.^10\,^20\,^40} \quad = 0.125$$

Try the others in Activity 9.2.

9	9	9	9	.	9	9	9
8	8	8	8	.	8	8	8
7	7	7	7	.	7	7	7
6	6	6	6	.	6	6	6
5	5	5	5	.	5	5	5
4	4	4	4	.	4	4	4
3	3	3	3	.	3	3	3
2	2	2	2	.	2	2	2
1	1	1	1	.	1	1	1
0	0	0	0	.	0	0	0
1000s	100s	10s	Units		1/10ths	1/100ths	1/1000ths

Figure 9.1: Fractions and decimals chart

Activity 9.2 — *Fractions and decimal equivalent*

Fraction	Division	Decimal equivalent
$\dfrac{6}{10}$		0.6
$\dfrac{2}{10}$		0.2
$\dfrac{9}{10}$		0.9
$\dfrac{4}{5}$		0.8
$\dfrac{3}{5}$		0.6
$\dfrac{3}{8}$		0.375
$\dfrac{7}{8}$		0.875
$\dfrac{7}{2}$		3.5
$\dfrac{25}{4}$		6.25

The answers to Activity 9.2 are given at the end of the chapter.

One more thing before we leave the chart. Sometimes, using the 1/10th column is still not small enough to get an accurate measurement. The numbers are, therefore, cut into even smaller pieces of ten each to give you 1/10th of 1/10th. This gives you the 1/100th column. Next to that there is a column for still smaller measurements (1/10th of 1/10th of 1/10th) or 1/1000th.

Last, a look at 0.25 (0 in the units column, 2 in the 1/10ths and 5 in the 1/100ths column). Note that this is the same as saying 25/100 or 25 for every hundred or 25 per hundred or 25 per cent (25%). So any decimal figure, say 0.38, translates immediately to 38/100 or 38%. The same thing applies to a single decimal figure such as 0.8. All you do is add a '0' to the '8' to bring it into the 1/100th column to make it 80/100 or 80%. Again, there is nothing to learn. Time for some practice. Have a go at converting some fractions to decimals and to percentages and the reverse in Activity 9.3.

Activity 9.3 — Converting fractions, decimals and percentages

Fractions to decimals

$\dfrac{1}{10}$ =

$\dfrac{3}{10}$ =

$\dfrac{4}{5}$ =

$\dfrac{6}{8}$ =

$\dfrac{25}{10}$ =

$\dfrac{4}{8}$ =

Decimals to fractions

0.25 =

0.6 =

0.4 =

0.15 =

1.5 =

1.2 =

Percentage to fraction to decimal

80% = =

50% = =

60% = =

25% = =

75% = =

12½% = =

Decimal to fraction to percentage

0.2 = =

0.8 = =

0.1 = =

0.5 = =

0.4 = =

0.12 = =

The answers to Activity 9.3 are given at the end of the chapter.

Conversions of weights and volumes

Let's move on to the next area of basic numeracy which is important for the test and also forms a part of many healthcare calculations. It is essential to be able to convert weights and volumes within the metric system. Fortunately it's easy as you generally only have to confront multiplying and dividing by 1000. For example, 1 litre is made up of 1000 millilitres ('milli' means 'a thousand') and 1 gramme (gram) is made up of 1000 milligrammes (milligrams). So, to convert 1 litre into millilitres you simply multiply by 1000; it's the same for 1 gram, to get 1000 milligrams. You can convert the 1000 millilitres and 1000 milligrams back again by dividing by 1000. Another way of looking at it is that 1 millilitre is 1/1000th of a litre and 1 milligram is 1/1000th of a gram. Have a look at Table 9.1.

The metric system
Weight is measured in kilograms (kg) Volume is measured in litres (l) Length is measured in metres (m) Amount of substance is measured in moles (mol)
Weight
e.g. the amount of a drug in a tablet such as frusemide 30mg tablets 1 gram (g) = 1/1000th of a kilogram 1 milligram (mg) = 1/1000th of a gram 1 microgram (mcg) = 1/1000th of a milligram 1 nanogram (ng) = 1/1000th of a microgram
Volume
e.g. the strength of a drug expressed as its weight in a given volume of a liquid, such as amoxicillin trihydrate, 125mg in 5ml of syrup 1 millilitre (ml) = 1/1000th of a litre 1 microlitre (mcl) = 1/1000th of a millilitre
Length
e.g. the diameter of an epithelial cell may be 120mcm 1 millimetre (mm) = 1/1000th of a metre 1 micrometre (mcm) = 1/1000th of a millimetre 1 nanometre (nm) = 1/1000th of a micrometre

Table 9.1: The metric system of measurement

To do conversions quickly and easily, most people use the 'bouncing decimal' or 'jumping rabbit' technique. If you look at Figure 9.1 again and find 1000 (and include the decimal point), all you need to do is bounce the decimal point three times to the left, over each '0' until you stop between the 1 in the thousands column and the '0' in the hundreds column:

1   .0   0   0.

1000s   100s   10s   units

You have now changed 1000 into 1.000 (or just 1) or 1000 milligrams (mg), say, into 1 gram (g). You do the same thing in the opposite direction to change 1g into 1000mg. Just bounce the decimal point three times to the right, starting with its position after the 1 in the units column and over each '0' until you stop after the 1/1000ths column:

1	.0	0	0 .
units	1/10ths	1/100ths	1/1000ths

You have now converted 1 (or 1.0) into 1000 or, say, 1g into 1000mg. The same movements apply to changing, say, 2.5g to milligrams (2500mg) or 0.5g to milligrams (500mg) and the reverse, say, 1500mg to grams (1.5g) or 250mg to grams (0.25g).

Remember, there will always be many more milligrams than grams, giving you a bigger number for your answer. The same applies to micrograms (mcg) compared with milligrams. There will always be more because they are much smaller. The same applies for millilitres (ml) compared with litres (l). Remember, too, the 'magic' number three is the number of times you move the decimal point. Try the conversions in Activity 9.4.

Activity 9.4 — Metric conversion

1.	2g	=	mg	10.	4000mcg	=	mg
2.	1.5g	=	mg	11.	2750mcg	=	mg
3.	0.75g	=	mg	12.	3500mcg	=	mg
4.	4500mg	=	g	13.	1L	=	ml
5.	375mg	=	g	14.	1.5L	=	ml
6.	30mg	=	g	15.	2.75L	=	ml
7.	1.5mg	=	mcg	16.	1000ml	=	l
8.	1.625mg	=	mcg	17.	1500ml	=	l
9.	3.055mg	=	mcg	18.	1250ml	=	l

The answers to Activity 9.4 are given at the end of the chapter.

Cancelling down and decimal equivalent

We've already had a look at finding the decimal equivalent of a fraction (Activity 9.2). Sometimes, though, the fraction might be a bit bigger so, before dividing the bottom into the top and to make your life easier, it can be simplified. (You will need this skill when doing even simple health-care calculations.)

For example: $\frac{16}{32}$ can be simplified to $\frac{1}{2}$

You may prefer to do this in stages. The trick is to find a number that will go into both the figure on the top of the fraction and the figure on the bottom. (It's a bit like cutting a grape in half and then an apple in half so that two people get an equal amount of grape and apple.) The figures in our fraction (16 and 32) can, likewise, be 'cut in half' or divided into two (they are both even numbers so they can be divided into equal parts by two):

$$\frac{16}{32} \boxed{2} = \frac{8}{16} \quad \text{Now divide by 2 again:} \quad \frac{8}{16} \boxed{2} = \frac{4}{8}$$

and again:

$$\frac{4}{8} \boxed{2} = \frac{2}{4}$$

and for the last time . . .

$$\frac{2}{4} \boxed{2} = \frac{1}{2}$$

You have now simplified

$$\frac{16}{32} \quad \text{to} \quad \frac{1}{2}$$

As for the decimal equivalent, you probably know that 1/2 is the same as 0.5 and you can prove it in the usual way, by dividing the bottom into the top:

$$\frac{1}{2} \uparrow \qquad \text{Set it out as usual:} \qquad 2 \overline{)1.^10} \quad = 0.5$$

(Always go up,
like the fountains in
Trafalgar Square)

Whilst on simplification of fractions, you will remember, perhaps, crossing off noughts (0s) to break down a fraction such as 100/1000 to 1/10 like this:

$$\frac{10\theta}{100\theta} = \frac{1\theta}{10\theta} = \frac{1}{10}$$

A word of warning, though. Don't be 'noughtist'. Don't cancel every nought you see. Remember, for each stage, cancel only one '0' off the top and one off the bottom, following the rule of 'doing the same to the top as you do to the bottom'. By the way, the result is the same as if you had divided both the top and the bottom by 10 (or moved the decimal point one place) and then repeated the process again to get to 1/10.

You also might like to remember that any figure ending in a '5', say, 125, will always divide by 5 and so will any figure ending in a '0', say 100. So, if you have a fraction of 100/125, you can cancel down in stages:

$$\frac{100}{125} \boxed{5} = \frac{20}{25} \boxed{5} = \frac{4}{5}$$

(Of course, you could have divided the top and the bottom by 25 to achieve the same result.)
And the decimal equivalent is . . .

$$\frac{0\,.\,8}{5\overline{)4\,.\,{}^{4}0}} \quad (0.8)$$

Try the examples in Activity 9.5.

Activity 9.5　　　　　　　　　　　　　*Cancelling down and decimal equivalent*

Cancel down the fraction	Division	Decimal equivalent
$\dfrac{3}{15}$		_____
$\dfrac{15}{25}$		_____
$\dfrac{4}{6}$		_____
$\dfrac{7}{28}$		_____
$\dfrac{25}{75}$		_____
$\dfrac{2}{10}$		_____
$\dfrac{120}{150}$		_____

The answers to Activity 9.5 are given at the end of the chapter.

Multiplying fractions

The next skill you will require for healthcare calculations (and therefore, probably for the test)
is that of multiplying fractions. You will need it, for example, when calculating the correct volume
of a fluid to be administered to a patient, by mouth or by injection, in order to give the correct
dose, according to the prescription. Like the other skills we've looked at, it just requires a basic

knowledge of what to do. You will know, for example, that a half of one is a half. This is the same as saying 'a half times one is a half' and you would set it out as follows:

$$\frac{1}{2} \times \frac{1}{1}$$

Put an extra '1' here to remind you to multiply the bottom as well as the top

Now multiply the top of the fraction and the bottom.

$$\frac{1}{2} \times \frac{1}{1} = \frac{1}{2}$$

So, we have proved that half of one is a half. Brilliant!

Let's do another one to which you will know the answer – a half of a half:

$$\frac{1}{2} \times \frac{1}{2} = \frac{1}{4}$$ And the decimal equivalent?

Here's another to which you might not know the answer – two-fifths of three-quarters:

$$\frac{2}{5} \times \frac{3}{4} = \frac{6}{20}$$ Now, cancel down: $\frac{6}{20} = \frac{3}{10}$ And the decimal equivalent?

Try the examples in Activity 9.6.

Activity 9.6   *Multiplying fractions*

$\dfrac{1}{2} \times \dfrac{1}{5}$ =   —   Decimal equivalent   _____

$\dfrac{3}{4} \times \dfrac{1}{2}$ =   —   Decimal equivalent   _____

$\dfrac{1}{6} \times \dfrac{3}{5}$ =   —   Decimal equivalent   _____

$\dfrac{2}{5} \times \dfrac{5}{4}$ =   —   Decimal equivalent   _____

$\dfrac{1}{10} \times \dfrac{3}{2}$ =   —   Decimal equivalent   _____

The answers to Activity 9.6 are given at the end of the chapter.

Percentages

Shops use percentages for marking discounts (such as '25% off all garden furniture this weekend'), employers for pay rises (if you're very lucky) and they are used in healthcare to indicate the strength of a solution. This is why some simple calculations using percentages may appear in your test. In all cases, the figure given is the amount out of a hundred (the amount per cent). So, 25 per cent (25%) means 25 out of a hundred. If the price of the table and chairs is £100, for example, you pay £75 (£100 less £25). The percentage 25% can also be shown as the fraction 25/100 and simplified to 1/4, the decimal equivalent of which is 0.25. You see how they are all connected? Have a look back at Figure 9.1 for help.

Continuing the theme, suppose you wanted to work out what you have to pay if the furniture originally cost £150. You would have to calculate 25% of (or 25/100 ×) 150 and you would set it out like this:

$$150 \times \frac{25}{100} = 150 \times \frac{\overset{1}{25}}{\underset{4}{\cancel{100}}} \qquad 4\overline{\smash{\big)}150.0}^{\,37.5} = £37.50$$

Now, take this away from the original price of £150 (150 – 37.5) and you have worked out what you need to pay: £112.50p

Check that this is correct by adding the two amounts (112.5 + 37.5 = 150).

Have a look at Activity 9.7.

Activity 9.7 — *Percentages*

Solve the following:

1. 80% of 300 _____
2. 50% of 630 _____
3. 60% of 250 _____
4. 15% of 580 _____
5. 12½% of 200 _____
6. 33⅓% of 900 (to the nearest 100) _____
7. 23.5% of 200 _____
8. 42% of 150 _____
9. 75% of 750 (to one decimal place) _____
10. 12% of 75 _____

The answers to Activity 9.7 are given at the end of the chapter.

Ratios

Like percentages, ratios are used in healthcare to give the strength of a solution. For example, if there is one part of solute to 1000ml of solution, the ratio is 1 : 1000. You may be more familiar, perhaps, with that moment after a meal with a friend at a restaurant, when the bill arrives. You'll probably agree to 'go halves' or 'go 50 : 50'. You understand that the money is to be split 'down the middle' or halved and that's what the ratio of 50 : 50 means. It is equal on both sides – the same as 25 : 25 or 1 : 1.

Ratios are also a way of establishing and comparing amounts. They are not, therefore, always equal, as in the example of the solution, above. For example, £250 is to be divided between two people in the ratio 2 : 3. To work this out, you need to add the ratio figures together (2 + 3 = 5) and divide this into 250 to find one share (250/5 = 50).

Multiply one share (50) by each of the ratio figures:

$(2 \times 50) = £100$
$(3 \times 50) = £150$ and the money is shared in the correct portions.

(Check that the total comes back to £250.)

You may well be asked to do some calculations like this for your test. Have a go at the two in Activity 9.8.

Activity 9.8   *Ratios*

1. 36 chocolates are to be shared between a student and lecturer in the ratio 4 : 5. How many does each have?

   Student_____ Lecturer_____

2. In a month, the radiography department has taken 1000 X-rays in the ratio 2 : 3 for men and women. How many men had X-rays?

   Men_____

The answers to Activity 9.8 are given at the end of the chapter.

You may also be asked just to simplify existing ratios and you can do this by dividing both sides by the same number. (Fractions are simplified in a similar way.)

For example,   25 : 30 (divide each by 5)   =   a ratio of 5 : 6

or   16 : 8 (divide each by 8)   =   a ratio of 2 : 1

Comparing ratios is also a little like comparing fractions. They have to be of the same type in order to compare them. For example, compare two glucose solutions of different strengths. One is mixed in the ratio of glucose to water of 1 : 20 and the other 2 : 38.

Multiply the first ratio by 2 so you can compare the two:

$1 : 20 \times 2 = 2 : 40$

This compares with the other solution at $2 : 38$, and it is clear now that this is the stronger solution (it contains less water).

You could, of course, have halved the second solution's ratio, making it $1 : 19$ and compared this with $1 : 20$. The answer is the same provided you compare like with like.

Have a look at Activity 9.9.

Activity 9.9   *Simplifying ratios*

Simplify the following ratios:

1. $12 : 2$ = _____

2. $100 : 1000$ = _____

3. $60 : 24$ = _____

4. $14 : 28$ = _____

5. Which group has more women in the following ratio of men to women:
     $1 : 6$ or $2 : 15$? _____

6. Which town has more cats in the ratio of dogs to cats of:
     $3 : 7$ or $6 : 12$? _____

The answers to Activity 9.9 are given at the end of the chapter.

Analogue to digital time

In the healthcare environment, the times when patients should receive their medication are expressed and noted down in digital time. Your test, therefore, may include conversions from normal (analogue) clock time to digital time and the reverse. If you look at the clock face below, the reason why digital timings are important becomes obvious. Can you read from the clock whether it is half past one in the morning (a.m.) or in the afternoon (p.m.)?

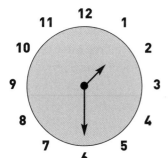

Any mistake is soon put right if only digital time is used, that is, either 01:30 or 13:30. Try Activity 9.10.

Activity 9.10   *Converting analogue to digital time and the reverse*

Analogue time   Digital time

1. 7.45 a.m.   _____

2. 7.45 p.m.   _____

3. 12.10 a.m.   _____

4. 12.10 p.m.   _____

Digital time   Analogue time

5. 18:35   _____

6. 22:20   _____

7. 03:45   _____

8. 11:05   _____

The answers to Activity 9.10 are given at the end of the chapter.

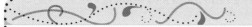

Chapter summary

Well, if you've managed to read this far, well done. Have a go at the specimen tests at the end of the chapter, which cover the areas we have looked at, and see how you get on. Don't forget to keep to the time limit. If you don't do as well as you thought you would, see which areas need revision and go back to the explanation in this chapter. Let's hope you do well. The test you sit on the day is bound to be different because it will be set out according to the preferences of the individual university and it may include areas not covered here. Most institutions, however, will provide a sample of their test before the day on their websites and if they don't, there's no harm in asking.

Here are a last few thoughts in case you are still feeling wobbly about numeracy. Much of life is about confidence, but before you can achieve that, you have to be competent. To be a concert pianist or a lead singer in a band, for example, you have to be competent in what you are doing. This will come with knowledge in the first place and practice thereafter and as painful as the hours of practice might be, you will finally grasp the success you deserve and become a confident performer. As some might say, 'no pain – no gain' and there really isn't anything satisfactory in gaining something if, on the way, it hasn't required some effort on your part. The question is, can we transfer these ideas to problems with numeracy? Can we gain the confidence which leads to that competence? To quote a number of luminaries, from Bob the Builder to Barack Obama, 'Yes we can!' (Actually it's 'Yes he can' for Bob the Builder, but let's not worry about that now.)

Further reading

Shihab, P (2009) *Numeracy in Nursing and Healthcare.* Harlow: Pearson.

Essentially a book on healthcare calculations but there are three chapters containing a good review of the basics.

Starkings, S and Krause, L (2015) *Passing Calculations Tests for Nursing Students*, 3rd edition. London: Sage/Learning Matters.

Healthcare calculations – useful introductory material.

Gatford, JD and Phillips NM (2011) *Nursing Calculations*, 8th edition. London: Churchill Livingstone.

Clearly laid out basic numeracy pages before continuing with healthcare calculations.

Perkins, AF (2014) *Making Friends with Numbers.* London: K.U. Press.

Basic numeracy for the very worried plus most healthcare calculations you will need for the course.

Useful websites

www.bbc.co.uk/skillswise

Basic numeracy only, including games which help familiarisation and speed.

www.bbc.co.uk/skillswise/topic/nursing-and-care

Explains why numeracy skills are important in nursing with some useful tests for you to practise your skills.

www.snap.nhs.uk

Useful revision material with areas specific to healthcare. Select the 'have a go' box to try it out.

Answers to activities

Activity 9.1 Adding, taking away, multiplying and dividing decimals

1.	19.5	7.	8.58
2.	63.28	8.	278.88
3.	2.15	9.	451.18
4.	4.71	10.	2.45
5.	29.99	11.	48.5
6.	10.27	12.	250.5

Activity 9.2 Fractions and decimal equivalent

Fraction	Division	Decimal equivalent

$\dfrac{6}{10}$ $\quad 10\overline{\smash{)}6.{}^60}$ with quotient 0.6 → 0.6

$\dfrac{2}{10}$ $\quad 10\overline{\smash{)}2.{}^20}$ with quotient 0.2 → 0.2

$\dfrac{9}{10}$ $\quad 10\overline{\smash{)}9.{}^90}$ with quotient 0.9 → 0.9

$\dfrac{4}{5}$ $\quad 5\overline{\smash{)}4.{}^40}$ with quotient 0.8 → 0.8

$\dfrac{3}{5}$ $\quad 5\overline{\smash{)}3.{}^30}$ with quotient 0.6 → 0.6

$\dfrac{3}{8}$ $\quad 8\overline{\smash{)}3.{}^30\,{}^60\,{}^40}$ with quotient 0.375 → 0.375

$\dfrac{7}{8}$ $\quad 8\overline{\smash{)}7.{}^70\,{}^60\,{}^40}$ with quotient 0.875 → 0.875

$\dfrac{7}{2}$ $\quad 2\overline{\smash{)}7.{}^10}$ with quotient 3.5 → 3.5

$\dfrac{25}{4}$ $\quad 4\overline{\smash{)}25.{}^10\,{}^20}$ with quotient 6.25 → 6.25

Activity 9.3 Converting fractions, decimals and percentages

Fractions to decimals			Decimals to fractions		
$\dfrac{1}{10}$	=	0.1	0.25	=	$\dfrac{1}{4}$
$\dfrac{3}{10}$	=	0.3	0.6	=	$\dfrac{3}{5}$
$\dfrac{4}{5}$	=	0.8	0.4	=	$\dfrac{2}{5}$
$\dfrac{6}{8}$	=	0.75	0.15	=	$\dfrac{3}{20}$
$\dfrac{25}{10}$	=	2.5	1.5	=	$1\dfrac{1}{2}$
$\dfrac{4}{8}$	=	0.5	1.2	=	$1\dfrac{1}{5}$

Percentage to fraction to decimal				Decimal to fraction to percentage			
80%	=	$\frac{4}{5}$	= 0.8	0.2	=	$\frac{1}{5}$	= 20%
50%	=	$\frac{1}{2}$	= 0.5	0.8	=	$\frac{4}{5}$	= 80%
60%	=	$\frac{3}{5}$	= 0.6	0.1	=	$\frac{1}{10}$	= 10%
25%	=	$\frac{1}{4}$	= 0.25	0.5	=	$\frac{1}{2}$	= 50%
75%	=	$\frac{3}{4}$	= 0.75	0.4	=	$\frac{2}{5}$	= 40%
12½%	=	$\frac{1}{8}$	= 0.125	0.12	=	$\frac{3}{25}$	= 12%

Activity 9.4 Metric conversions

1.	2000mg	7.	1500mcg	13.	1000ml
2.	1500mg	8.	1625mcg	14.	1500ml
3.	750mg	9.	3055mcg	15.	2750ml
4.	4.5g	10.	4mg	16.	1l
5.	0.375g	11.	2.75mg	17.	1.5l
6.	0.03g	12.	3.5mg	18.	1.25l

Activity 9.5 Cancelling down and decimal equivalent

Cancel down the fraction	Division	Decimal equivalent
$\frac{3}{15} = \frac{1}{5}$	$5\,)\overline{1.0}$ — 0.2	0.2
$\frac{15}{25} = 3$	$5\,)\overline{3.0}$ — 0.6	0.6
$\frac{4}{6} = \frac{2}{3}$	$3\,)\overline{2.000}$ — 0.666	0.67 (to 2 decimal places)
$\frac{7}{8} = \frac{1}{4}$	$4\,)\overline{1.00}$ — 0.25	0.25
$\frac{25}{75} = \frac{1}{3}$	$3\,)\overline{1.000}$ — 0.333	0.33 (to 2 decimal places)
$\frac{2}{10} = \frac{1}{5}$	$5\,)\overline{1.0}$ — 0.2	0.2
$\frac{120}{150} = \frac{4}{5}$	$5\,)\overline{4.0}$ — 0.8	0.8

Activity 9.6 Multiplying fractions

				Decimal equivalent	0.1

$$\frac{1}{2} \times \frac{1}{5} = \frac{1}{10}$$ Decimal equivalent   0.1

$$\frac{3}{4} \times \frac{1}{2} = \frac{3}{8}$$ Decimal equivalent   0.375

$$\frac{1}{6} \times \frac{3}{5} = \frac{3}{30} \quad \frac{(1)}{(10)}$$ Decimal equivalent   0.1

$$\frac{2}{5} \times \frac{5}{4} = \frac{10}{20} \quad \frac{(1)}{(2)}$$ Decimal equivalent   0.5

$$\frac{1}{10} \times \frac{3}{2} = \frac{3}{20}$$ Decimal equivalent   0.15

Activity 9.7 Percentages

1. 240
2. 315
3. 150
4. 87
5. 25
6. 300
7. 47
8. 63
9. 562.5
10. 9

Activity 9.8 Ratios

1. Student: 16

   Lecturer: 20
2. 400 (women: 600)

Activity 9.9 Simplifying ratios

1. 6 : 1
2. 1 : 10
3. 5 : 2
4. 1 : 2
5. 2 : 15
6. 3 : 7

Activity 9.10 Converting analogue to digital time and the reverse

Digital time	Analogue time
1. 07:45	5. 6:35 p.m.
2. 19:45	6. 10:20 p.m.
3. 00:10	7. 3:45 a.m.
4. 12:10	8. 11:05 a.m.

Specimen paper 1

This paper has 25 questions
Time allowed: 25 minutes
Calculators are <u>not</u> permitted

Name_____

Solve the following:

Use this space for your workings

1. $12.9 + 8.7$ =

2. $0.6 + 2.65$ =

3. $67.8 - 38.9$ =

4. $2.8 - 1.94$ =

5. 13.4×27.8 =

6. 80.5×3.04 =

7. $58.14 \div 1.7$ =

8. $1770.72 \div 5.1$ =

Convert to decimals:

9. $\dfrac{9}{10}$ =

10. $\dfrac{7}{8}$ =

Convert to *simple* fractions:

11. 0.3 =

12. 0.125 =

Convert the following:

13. $1.7g$ = mg

14. $250mg$ = g

Solve the following:

Use this space for your workings

15. 50% of 350 =

16. 18% of 490 =

Convert the following:

17. $\dfrac{4}{5}$ to a percentage =

18. 0.15 to a percentage =

Solve the following and give as your answer the *decimal equivalent*:

19. $\dfrac{1}{2} \times \dfrac{3}{4}$ =

20. $\dfrac{1}{4} \times \dfrac{1}{2}$ =

Cancel down the following and give as your answer the *decimal equivalent*:

21. $\dfrac{16}{64}$ =

Simplify the ratio:

22. 15 : 5 =

23. £75 is to be shared between 2,
    in the ratio of 3 : 2.
    How much is each given?
    =

Convert the following:

24. 1:25 a.m. to digital time =

25. 22:50 to analogue time =

End of test

Specimen paper 2

This paper has 25 questions
Time allowed: 25 minutes
Calculators are <u>not</u> permitted

Name_____

Solve the following:

Use this space for your workings

1. $24.9 + 16.7 \quad =$

2. $5.28 + 0.72 \quad =$

3. $58.6 - 23.9 \quad =$

4. $3.4 - 1.53 \quad =$

5. $22.2 \times 11.4 \quad =$

6. $42.5 \times 58.7 \quad =$

7. $129.6 \div 2.4 \quad =$

8. $551.52 \div 3.6 \quad =$

Convert to decimals:

9. $\frac{7}{10} \quad =$

10. $\frac{3}{8} \quad =$

Convert to *simple* fractions:

11. $0.2 \quad =$

12. $0.025 \quad =$

Convert the following:

13. $1.3g \quad = \quad mg$

14. $2.55mg \quad = \quad mcg$

Solve the following:

15. 50% of $750 \quad =$

16. 35% of $165 \quad =$

Convert the following:

17. $\frac{3}{5}$ to a percentage $\quad =$

18. 0.35 to a percentage $\quad =$

Solve the following and give as your answer the *decimal equivalent*:

19. $\frac{1}{2} \times \frac{1}{1} \quad =$

20. $\frac{1}{2} \times \frac{1}{2} \quad =$

Cancel down the following and give as your answer the *decimal equivalent*:

21. $\frac{20}{60} \quad =$

Simplify the ratio:

22. 12 : 4 =

23. £36 is to be shared between 2,

in the ratio of 4 : 5.

How much is each given?

=

Convert the following:

24. 7:15 a.m. to digital time   =

25. 21:25 to analogue time   =

Specimen paper 1: answers

1. 21.6	**13.** 1700mg
2. 3.25	**14.** 0.25g
3. 28.9	**15.** 175
4. 0.86	**16.** 88.2
5. 372.52	**17.** 80%
6. 244.72	**18.** 15%
7. 34.2	**19.** 0.375
8. 347.2	**20.** 0.125
9. 0.9	**21.** 0.25
10. 0.875	**22.** 3 : 1
11. $\dfrac{3}{10}$	**23.** 45/30
	24. 01:25
	25. 10:50 p.m.
12. $\dfrac{1}{8}$	

Specimen paper 2: answers

1. 41.6	**13.** 1300mg
2. 6	**14.** 2550mcg
3. 34.7	**15.** 375
4. 1.87	**16.** 57.75
5. 253.08	**17.** 60%
6. 2494.75	**18.** 35%
7. 54	**19.** 0.5
8. 153.2	**20.** 0.25
9. 0.7	**21.** 0.33
10. 0.375	**22.** 3 : 1
11. $\dfrac{1}{5}$	**23.** 16/20
	24. 07:15
	25. 9:25 p.m.
12. $\dfrac{1}{40}$	

Chapter 10
Literacy tests

Mandy Gough and Karen Elcock

Chapter aims

The aim of this chapter is for you to understand the importance of possessing strong literacy skills in nursing and how you can prepare for the literacy tests that you may encounter on your selection day.

By the end of this chapter you will be able to:

- understand what is meant by literacy, the skills it covers and its relevance for nursing;
- appreciate how poor literacy poses a risk to patients;
- understand how universities may assess your literacy skills at selection days;
- recognise your own personal strengths and areas for development in literacy and know where to go and who to ask to develop your skills further.

Introduction

The focus in this chapter is on literacy as it relates to English-language skills for adults. In fact, literacy today has a far wider meaning than it did, because the world has changed substantially in the last couple of decades: we are deeply engaged in the fast-moving digital age. Previously, we relied on more traditional forms of information and literacy was mostly being able to read and write. Nowadays, literacy both at work and at home takes on a far wider meaning, as information is transferred in many different forms. We now exchange information by text, visuals, video and audio, using a variety of tools: phones, text messaging and computers. It is not just the tools that change: language changes too and can influence writing and communication styles.

The UK is a multicultural society and as a result the English language itself is ever-changing, in both written and verbal formats. As a nurse you will encounter colleagues and patients who speak different kinds of English and as a nurse you are required to engage and make yourself understood and facilitate communication with everyone you meet, whether in written or spoken form. The Nursing and Midwifery Council (NMC) makes this very clear in the *Standards for Pre-registration Nursing Education* (Nursing and Midwifery Council, 2010), which state that:

All nurses must:

- *use a range of communication skills and technologies to support person-centred care and enhance quality and safety;*
- *ensure people receive all the information they need in a language and manner that allow them to make informed choices and share decision making;*
- *recognise when language interpretation or other communication support is needed and know how to obtain it;*
- *use the full range of communication methods, including verbal, non-verbal and written, to acquire, interpret and record their knowledge and understanding of people's needs;*
- *be aware of their own values and beliefs and the impact this may have on their communication with others;*
- *take account of the many different ways in which people communicate and how these may be influenced by ill health, disability and other factors, and be able to recognise and respond effectively when a person finds it hard to communicate.*

Therefore when considering literacy we cannot see it as one skill alone: it is interlinked with other skills such as speaking, listening, reading and body language, gestures and expression. It is intertwined with social and cultural values. It is about communicating with others all the time, finding ways to overcome barriers, using not just traditional methods but also up-to-date 'literacies'.

What is literacy?

Before you skip this chapter indignantly, saying 'I don't need help with literacy', take a moment to consider two meanings of the word:

1. able to read and write: *their parents were uneducated and barely literate;*
2. having education or knowledge, typically in a specified area: *we need people who are economically and politically literate* (**http://oxforddictionaries.com**).

We can see the first meaning is the ability to read and write, and refers solely to the written word. The second meaning is more specialised: the word 'literate' (or 'literacy') is prefixed by adjectives: 'politically literate', 'economically literate'. Such phrases are examples of how language develops over time. While this chapter focuses on the written form of literacy, these other types of literacy are also needed in our everyday lives, at work and at university.

For example, nurses need to be computer-literate to keep up to date professionally, as so much information is online. In addition computers are increasingly used now for patient records rather than using written formats and patients are increasingly using computers to record data on their condition at home and upload it to their local GP practice. The term 'literacy' not only applies to pen and paper: how mobile phone-literate are you? How good are you at keeping within the word limit of a Tweet? The ability to paraphrase and summarise is essential if you are to use these tools, and they are the very same skills that you will need when studying and when at work.

It is not only about writing – it can be quite a skill to read from different formats. Reading relates not only to books but also, increasingly, to electronic devices such as computers, smartphones or an e-book reader. We are expected to read and understand a range of different types of texts and graphics. In nursing you will need to evaluate and interpret information quickly from a wide range of sources, and accuracy in doing so is essential. Evaluating information is also a skill required when writing and you will be expected to evaluate books, articles and research when writing your assignments. This may often start with a reflection on your own skills and attributes on commencing the course. Reflection, evaluation and critical thinking are closely related skills, all of which will require a certain level of literacy if you are to make your meaning clear.

Why is literacy important in nursing?

Chapter 9 highlighted the very significant risks we pose to patients if we use numerals incorrectly. The same risks exist when we consider our use of English. Accurately written records are essential in nursing. It is how we record what we have done for patients and also what further care they may need. Poor grammar or spelling, in particular, could mean that patients do not receive the care they need or worse, are given incorrect care. For example if you spelt a drug incorrectly, Carbimazole used for hyperthyroidism instead of Carbamazepine used for epileptic seizures, this could result in the patient receiving inappropriate care, which could have serious consequences. Also, as more patients are willing to complain about their care, accurate and legible record keeping is essential if you are to defend yourself when a complaint is made.

The following are excerpts from medical records and classic examples of poorly written English.

- The patient has no previous history of suicides.

- She is numb from her toes down.

- Patient was alert and unresponsive.

- Patient has two teenage children, but no other abnormalities (Lederer, 2002).

At first glance we may interpret these errors as being a result of poor writing, but it is also worth considering where the error started. For example, did the original speaker say the sentence incorrectly? Did the listener mishear? Was the original sentence written in notes so the person transcribing merely copied out word for word? Or did the writer misread the original sentence? Either way the writer did not really think about what they were writing.

The Nursing and Midwifery Council Code (**www.nmc-uk.org**) and Guidance on record keeping (NMC, 2009) make clear the importance of keeping accurate records with the latter document stating that:

> *Your records should be accurate and recorded in such a way that the meaning is clear.*

> *Records should be factual and not include unnecessary abbreviations, jargon, meaningless phrases or irrelevant speculation.*
> (NMC, 2009, p5)

A group of first-year nursing students were asked to consider the various meanings of literacy after their first placement experience and this is what they said:

Students' view . . . Literacy is:

more than just words;

the ability to use all the skills available, including reading, writing, speaking and listening. These may include pictures or sign language;

expressing yourself to someone to enable that person to understand what you are saying. It is also the ability to identify, understand, interpret, create and communicate;

the ability to express thoughts, feelings, ideas . . . a key piece of helping people to achieve their goals and develop their knowledge and potential and fully participate in society;

a form of communication . . . through telling a story about something to someone. Also a recording of true events, for example a historical happening, a conversation that you may have had with a patient.

Skills in practice	Skills at university
Patient records, care plans, patient notes, medication charts, assessment tools	Researching journals, books, reports
Handover reports	Lecturer-produced notes/handouts
Notes from telephone calls, conversations and observations	Blogs, e-mails, using websites
Patient referral and discharge letters/summaries	Essays, reports and exams
Notices, policies, updates	Presentations
Information leaflets for patients	Notes in lectures
Court reports	Portfolios, practice logs and reflective diaries

Table 10.1: Activities that require reading and writing skills

Table 10.1 includes some of the tasks and activities that require reading and/or writing skills in practice and at university.

As you can see, there is a wide range of activities where literacy will be important if you are to communicate with others clearly and effectively. Your course will help you become familiar with them.

Activity 10.1   *Everyday reading and writing*

Think about the reading and writing you do in your everyday life and make a list. What methods do you use most? When writing, who are you writing to/for?

In your list you will probably include writing e-mails and texts to friends. This is a very informal type of writing, where shortened and abbreviated forms are common and avoiding grammatical errors is not such a priority. They will also contain colloquial expressions and possibly language and symbols which would be deemed unacceptable in a formal context.

At university and in practice you are required to use more formal language, with the exception of notes that you may make for your own use. Notes at work comprise key words and may not be full sentences. Shortened forms and acronyms are acceptable as long as they are common words in your chosen field.

In contrast, essays are examples of formal academic writing with a specific structure. They must be written in full sentences and with no abbreviations. Acronyms can be used, but only after they have been written in full at first use. It is essential to conform to referencing protocols to show that work is evidence-based.

If you are looking at Table 10.1 and thinking that you have no idea of how to write in all these different ways, especially the more formal and specialised genres, do not panic. Universities will be looking for students who can show a good basic use of English; part of doing a degree is learning how to develop your academic writing skills.

What level of English do I need to get onto a nursing programme?

Entry requirements, in general, are that a prospective candidate should have a minimum of level 2 in English. In practice, this means a GCSE grade A–C in English or equivalent. Even if you have a certificate showing that you have achieved this level, you will still be required by most universities to sit a literacy test on selection day. This part of the selection process will most likely focus on both reading and writing skills.

It is worth noting that, while a level 2 standard of English is a sufficient minimum standard to gain entry, the demands of a degree course will require you to develop English skills above this level. This can present a challenge to many applicants, as during the course you will be expected to produce academic writing and read academic research.

The NMC is clear that the level of English required for entry to a pre-registration programme is a starting point and there needs to be a commitment from the student to develop these skills to proficiency during the course of the programme.

Types of literacy test

The literacy test is not a test of your nursing knowledge. The aims of literacy tests for entry onto a nursing degree are for you to show that you can:

- read, and demonstrate understanding of, a written task;
- complete a written task within a given time;

- write legibly;
- construct clear sentences and paragraphs;
- use grammar and punctuation correctly;
- spell accurately.

Literacy tests are likely to comprise one or more of the following:

- a short essay in response to a given title, which may be given in advance;
- a short essay reflecting on your contribution to a group exercise undertaken on the same day;
- multiple choice questions assessing understanding after reading a piece of text;
- a gap-fill exercise requiring you to insert the correct word into gaps in a text, usually from a set of words provided, to test grammar;
- questions asking you to read a piece of text and identify specific grammatical or spelling errors in it;
- responses to questions usually requiring the circling of a correct word spelling or synonym, or punctuating a sentence;
- a summarising or paraphrasing exercise;
- oral interview where speaking and listening may be assessed.

Students applying for a postgraduate pre-registration nursing programme may be asked to undertake a different type of literacy test to demonstrate their ability to undertake postgraduate level study, e.g. a critical appraisal of a short piece of research.

The pass mark will vary between universities and this information should be available to you on request. Many universities will send you a sample of the test with your invitation to attend your interview or direct you to their website where sample tests are available.

Activity 10.2   *Literacy tests*

Google the term '**nursing literacy tests:ac.uk**'. Among the results will be university websites with sample literacy tests (some also provide answers as well!). Look at the tests that different universities use. Try them out and, if possible, ask someone who is good at English to look at your answers to give you feedback. If you find you have problems in specific areas, or in completing the papers in general, refer to the websites and recommended books at the end of this chapter, which can help you improve your literacy skills.

We will now look at some of these formats along with the specific language skills they aim to test.

The essay

This is usually a free-writing question where you are asked to write about a given topic, such as:

- Why is the ability to write good English in nursing important?

- Why is communication important in nursing?

- Write about a situation where you gave someone bad news.

Or you may take part in a group discussion and then be asked to write about your contribution to the discussion. This requires you to be honest about what you did well and what you could have improved on. Don't be worried about writing about any of your weaknesses, this will be seen as a positive, as it demonstrates self-awareness which is important in nursing.

You will be told whether there is a word limit; on average it is 150–200 words, or they may ask for a set number of sentences or pages. You will be given a set time in which to do this, such as 10 minutes for 150–200 words. If there are several parts to a test then a specific period of time may be given for all components of the test, in which case it is expected that you manage the time appropriately so that you can complete all sections. Time management is an important skill in work and study and you may find that this is an area being assessed in another part of the interview. You should find out beforehand if the writing is done on a keyboard or by hand. If by hand, some marks may be awarded for legibility.

Marking will focus both on the mechanics of the writing and the content: they will want to see that you have understood what is required and that any views expressed are compatible with those expected of a nurse. When marking your essay they will look for the following points.

- The look and length of the text – if you write 50 words instead of 150 this will attract a lower mark. Does the response address the title? Is there a sense of a beginning, middle and end? Is it set out in appropriate paragraphs?

- The flow: can the reader easily follow what you are saying, e.g. are sentences well-formed, varied in length and linked using appropriate words?

- A range of vocabulary and tenses are used which are correctly spelled and grammatically formed. For example, are you using past tense when talking about the past? Have you used the correct ending?

- Punctuation: are basic punctuation marks, commas, full stops and apostrophes placed correctly?

- Spelling: are everyday words spelled correctly? Do not use text speak, e.g. 2, thnx, c u, ta.

- Writing style: is there an attempt to use more formal writing?

In summary, you will need to be able to express yourself:

- clearly;

- logically;

- objectively;

- succinctly;

- correctly.

You will always need to show that you can write in a way that the recipient can understand.

> Lecturer's tip . . . Practise short pieces of writing – take a topic that is in the news and turn it into your own essay question. As you are writing, remember to follow the advice above.
>
> Remember that this is not an English literature exam. In other words, you are not writing a novel, which usually contains a lot of descriptive adjectives; keep to the facts.

Reading and comprehension

The focus here is your ability to demonstrate that you can read and understand a short piece of text. This is often assessed using multiple choice questions or writing a summary from the text or short article you are given. The text may have line numbers to which they refer (see Activity 10.4 for an example). A multiple choice test will give you a choice of answers to questions about the text. They may ask you to choose the closest meaning to a specific sentence or paragraph or ask which line has a spelling mistake in it, or explain the meaning of a word that is used in the text.

Practising timed exercises and short essays will give you a better chance of completing all the questions in the test within the allotted time. There are numerous websites you can use to practise multiple choice test techniques, but also look at example test papers on university websites.

Comprehension involves understanding the whole text, its purpose and meaning as well as smaller parts, such as sentences and words. The examples below are typical of questions that may be asked after you have read the provided text.

1. The style of writing is best described as:

   a. informative   b. persuasive   c. entertaining   d. technical

2. Which word has the same meaning as 'contemporary'?

   a. futuristic   b. reproduction   c. current   d. fashionable

3. The main purpose of the e-mail is:

   a. to complain   b. to compliment   c. to invite   d. to inform

If you are asked to write a summary of a piece of text the intention is that you will not copy words directly from the text, but instead summarise the ideas in your own words. You can use key words or phrases, but must not copy whole sentences. The aim is to paraphrase (put into your own words) leaving out any specific examples or quotes they may use. To summarise a piece of text, read through the text first to get the main points then read through again highlighting key points. Use your own words to link these key points together.

Activity 10.3   *Summarising*

Summarise the following text:

The Francis report (2013) has had a significant impact on health care. For nursing a key area has been around the recruitment of nurses. One of the recommendations from Francis was the implementation of values-based recruitment by universities (e.g. multiple mini interviews or situational judgement tests) in the selection of candidates for pre-registration nursing programmes.

An outline answer to Activity 10.3 is given at the end of the chapter.

Grammar

Grammar is often tested in one paper together with spelling and punctuation. Grammar is about how language works; it is a set of rules about how sentences are constructed.

In short, it is the backbone of language and strictly speaking includes punctuation, although most people when asked for an example of grammar will say 'verbs', 'nouns' and 'adjectives'. These are parts of speech and they include:

- noun;
- pronoun;
- verb;
- adjective;
- adverb;
- preposition;
- conjunction;
- article.

If you are unsure of what any of these terms mean or how to use them, then look at the Word Grammar section on the BBC Skillswise website (**www.bbc.co.uk/skillswise/english**).

Other terms that would be useful to know are:

- synonyms: words with similar meanings;
- antonyms: words with opposite meanings;
- homographs: words that have the same spelling but are usually pronounced differently, e.g. to row a boat/they had a row;
- homophones: words that have the same pronunciation but different meanings: right/write, there/their;

- heteronyms: words with the same spelling but different meanings, e.g. a desert in Africa/to desert (leave) (remember a dessert is a pudding, however);
- passive verb: no information on who did the action: the window was broken;
- active verb: the person who did the action is given: the burglar broke the window.

Knowing the names of parts of speech is helpful as often feedback on written work from lecturers may comment on a specific speech part. It will also help you to identify which areas you need to revise. Additionally you may come across multiple choice questions which ask you to identify an adverb or noun (Activity 10.4).

Activity 10.4　　　　**Which of these sentences contains a passive verb?**

a. Finally, I had done it.

b. It took me a long time, but I did it.

c. Finishing it made my day.

d. Finally, it was finished.

The answer to Activity 10.4 is given at the end of the chapter.

Errors are frequently made with word order in a sentence, subject and verb agreement and use of articles and prepositions.

Gap questions

These can be used to test your grammar and will ask you to complete a sentence from a choice of words. For example:

1. Appropriately select from **they're**, **there** or **their** in each of the gaps in this sentence. .... are many students who meet with .... personal tutor just to check that .... covering the right areas in .... assignment.
2. .... students live in university accommodation than 10 years ago.

   (a) Few
   (b) Fewer
   (c) Less

The answers are given at the end of the chapter.

Punctuation

Punctuation is important as it makes written text easier to understand and read. The emphasis, intonation, pauses and rhythm that you use when you speak can only be made clear to a reader by using punctuation. If used incorrectly, the meaning of a sentence can be changed completely. For example:

There was one difficulty: only Ben knew the route to the cinema.

There was one difficulty only, Ben knew: the route to the cinema.

Punctuation is often assessed through reading of a piece of text which has punctuation missing (usually apostrophes, commas and full stops), and then being asked a series of multiple choice questions where you identify which line the errors are in (Activity 10.5).

Activity 10.5   *Health and safety regulations*

Swimmers must use the footbath before entering the swimming pool.   Line 1

Showers must be used when leaving the pool.   Line 2

Swimmers belongings must not be left at the poolside.   Line 3

Children under six years old must be accompanied.   Line 4

There is a missing apostrophe on . . .

a. Line 1   b. Line 2   c. Line 3   d. Line 4

The answer is given at the end of the chapter.

You should at a minimum revise the correct use of commas, full stops, colons and semicolons; these are where the most common errors arise. Apostrophes cause even more problems, especially deciding when to use it's or its. The simple answer is that it's is short for it is or it has, so:

It's a lovely day (it is)

It's been raining (it has)

In contrast, its is used to denote possession, so:

The book has lost its cover.

Lynne Truss's book *Eats, Shoots and Leaves* is an entertaining way to learn about punctuation (see Further reading, below).

Spelling

Spelling will be assessed in any free-writing exercise and may also be part of a multiple choice test.

1. Men and women should be cared for in _____ bays on the wards.

    (a) seperate

    (b) separate

    (c) separete

    (d) seperete

The answer is given at the end of the chapter.

If spelling is an area that concerns you, then practice is important. *Chambers Adult Learners' Guide to Spelling* (see Further reading) provides lots of useful tips for helping you to improve your spelling.

- Break the word into small chunks (cup and board for cupboard).
- Use more than one of your senses (read it, say it, use magnetic letters to make it).
- Use different levels of memory (by using different ways of learning and memorising a word).
- Practise regularly.
- Draw pictures in your mind of words (e.g. a bra in a li**bra**ry).
- Look at the shapes that words make.

Make a note of words as you go along. Be methodical. Ask others to help you. Rather than endlessly reading through lists of words, try to interact more. Ask a friend to take a correct spelling list and change each word so it is incorrectly spelled. Analyse your own errors; are certain word patterns more difficult? Do you have trouble with knowing when to use double letters? Do pairs of vowels cause a problem? Once you have identified common areas, make a point of searching for more words which follow the same pattern. Write them out and focus on learning them. Use a computer or mobile creatively: make your own crosswords, word puzzles and activities. Search out free programs such as **www.puzzlemaker.com** and develop your own puzzles with words you find difficult. Think about words that sound the same but have a different purpose or meaning in a sentence, for example, 'there' and 'their' or 'practise' and 'practice'.

Preparing for your test

Follow the tips and practice notes in this chapter. Use the Further reading section and websites at the end of this chapter to help you become familiar with test formats and also to improve your language and literacy skills. Books on grammar and punctuation have become very popular, even bestsellers, and are very readable. They are therefore a good place to start if you want to improve your English writing; some recent ones appear in the Further reading list, below. You will also find it useful to read up on current topics in nursing and healthcare as essay topics may focus on these. Journals such as *Nursing Times* or the *Nursing Standard* are good for current issues.

Academic English

Once you are at university you will be expected to write in an academic style. Guidelines will be available to explain the university's expectations and protocols. Academic writing is a subject in its own right and, as with other subjects, this is a skill that you will develop whilst studying. There will be guidance and support available, but as a higher education student you will be expected to take responsibility for identifying and developing skills that need further work.

Most universities deliver academic writing skills sessions and/or have academic writing workshops or advice desks. It is beyond the scope of this chapter to cover academic writing, but there is a plethora of books and online resources available which provide a great deal of guidance. It would be advisable to start work on developing your academic skills prior to your course and a starting point is to start reading. You should regularly read professional journals such as the *Nursing Standard, Nursing Times,* books and health-related websites. Note the style of writing, how words and grammar are used and how succinctly the author writes. Note how words are used to introduce topics and create arguments within a text. Read a paragraph, then cover the text and start writing it out in your own words. Get into the habit of summarising a text, a film or a live event. Reading is the best way to learn how to write, but be choosy about what you read. Try to focus on evidence-based texts as opposed to lengthy novels. The more you read the more you will increase your vocabulary and skills at writing.

Tips for reading

A useful skill to acquire is the ability to 'read' through a book quickly to identify whether it meets your needs and identify the key points it is making.

- Take clues from the title – is it relevant? What do I expect the text to answer?
- Note the text structure – layout, paragraphs, topic sentences and conclusions.
- Scan through chapters for specific information to find key information quickly. Skim through the text to get the main ideas to gain an overall understanding. Read the first sentence of each paragraph. Read the first and last paragraphs of a chapter.

> Lecturer tip ... Keep a notebook and write down key points, or summarise important chapters into a couple of paragraphs. Note down words you don't know when reading and look them up later.

What to do if you're worried about your literacy skills

If you are still concerned about your ability to pass the literacy test, have dyslexia or have already failed the test at universities you have applied for, there are still some options.

If you have been diagnosed as dyslexic, contact the admissions team and the disability team at the university before your interview and let them know as you may be eligible for reasonable adjustments such as extra time and your dyslexia will need to be taken into account. In addition it is important that when you have been accepted at your chosen university that you make contact with the disability team there before starting so that they can start to look at the support you will need while you are on your course.

Go to Learn Direct (**www.learndirect.co.uk**) or visit the Move On website to find out about courses to improve your English writing. These are short courses and may be free for you to use depending on your qualifications and circumstances. Also talk to the admissions team at the universities you are interested in; some offer short courses in English to help applicants.

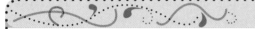

Chapter summary

The ability to communicate with patients, colleagues and the people you will come into contact with at work and in the university is an essential skill in nursing. Without this skill patient safety and the quality of care they receive are put at risk. The focus in this chapter has been on literacy as written English, which is just one of the many forms of communication that you will use on the programme. English writing skills are also essential for writing assignments and therefore being successful in your studies; if this is an area that concerns you, then preparation is essential. Remember, once you are on a course your university will provide support to help you develop your academic skills.

Further reading

Betteridge, A (2011) *Chambers Adult Learners' Guide to Spelling.* London: Chambers Harrap.
A practical guide to spelling which has also been approved by the British Dyslexia Association.

Giminez, J (2011) *Writing for Nursing and Midwifery Students*, 2nd edition. Basingstoke: Palgrave Macmillan.
A really useful book to equip you with the skills for academic writing.

Taggart, C and Wines, J (2011) *My Grammar and I (Or Should That Be 'Me'?): Old-school ways to sharpen your English.* London: Michael O'Mara Books.
An amusing but really helpful book on English grammar.

Truss, L (2009) *Eats, Shoots and Leaves.* London: Profile Books.
Another amusing book that teaches you about punctuation.

Useful websites

The following websites are all are aimed at helping people improve their reading, writing and grammar skills. Most have quizzes and tests so that you can check out which areas you need to improve upon and how you are improving.

http://englishforuniversity.com
Aimed at international students.

http://oxforddictionaries.com

Lots of useful tips and tests.

www.bbc.co.uk/schools/ks2bitesize/english

Aimed at children but fun.

www.bbc.co.uk/skillswise/english

Aimed at adults.

www.englishgrammar.org

English Grammar looks at both how English grammar is constructed and the areas where many people make mistakes.

Answers to activities and sample questions

Activity 10.3

In response to the Francis Report (2013) universities now use values-based recruitment to select student nurses.

Activity 10.4

The answer is (d): Finally, it was finished.

Gap questions

1. There, their, they're, their.

2. (b) Fewer.

Activity 10.5

The correct answer is (c), line 3.

Spelling

The correct answer is (b), separate.

Chapter 11
The selection day

Beattie Dray

Chapter aims

This chapter explores the many different ways that applicants are selected for a nursing degree programme. By the end of this chapter you will:

- have an insight into the different approaches used by universities to select candidates;
- understand the values and qualities that universities are looking for;
- be able to prepare for the different selection approaches used;
- gain an insight into the mistakes made by candidates at selection days and learn how to avoid them.

Introduction

The biggest fear for applicants is the unknown, the 'what ifs'. What if they ask me a question I can't answer? What if something happens that I'm totally unprepared for?

One of the problems for applicants is that each university uses different approaches to selection. You might go to one university and have just a group discussion and then to another where you have a traditional face-to-face interview.

That is why this chapter uses the word 'selection' rather than 'interview'. It may be that you won't have a traditional face-to-face interview, so you need to be prepared for all the different approaches that universities use to select candidates for their courses. The activities in this chapter will help you identify the different skills and attributes you have that the universities will be looking for at your selection day. You may also find them helpful in preparing your personal statement for your UCAS application if you have not already written it.

Situational tests

Before looking at the actual selection day it is worth mentioning that some universities now require students they have shortlisted to undertake an online test, usually at home, which they have to pass before being invited to attend their selection day. These are called situational tests or situational judgment tests. They are multiple choice questions based on a scenario which are used to test your knowledge, abilities, attitudes and personality traits to ensure that you possess the right characteristics for nursing. There are some examples of these tests on the internet if you Google for them which will give you an idea what to expect, and a link at the end of the chapter.

The format of the day

The format of the day will vary from university to university with the selection process taking anything from a half to a whole day. At a minimum there will be a presentation about the programme from academic staff who deliver it, along with an opportunity to ask questions and some type of face-to-face engagement with candidates, e.g. an interview or group activities.

Some universities will also give a tour of the campus, but others may not, so where a tour is not on offer it is worth finding out about and arranging to attend an open day so that you can get a real feel of the university.

An increasing number of universities have introduced numeracy and literacy tests for candidates regardless of their entry qualifications. In many cases such tests will take place in the first part of the day with only those candidates who meet the required level progressing to the next part of the selection day. We looked at numeracy and literacy in Chapters 9 and 10, so refer back if you need help with these areas.

How to find out which selection method a university uses

You will be sent information giving the format of the selection day in the letter/e-mail inviting you to attend. There may also be information available on the university website about what you can expect and many also tell you what they expect from you, which can help in your preparations for the day. Remember to confirm your attendance and if any problems arise that prevent you from attending, contact them and let them know.

There are many internet discussion forums where students talk about their selection day experiences, which can give you further insights. We gave details of some of these websites in Chapter 7.

Many of these discussion forums will give lists of questions that previous candidates have been asked or examples of group activities or scenarios used. There are, however, problems in relying on this kind of information: first, the information might be out of date and second, preparing answers to questions you think you will be asked can lead to further problems. Universities do realise that applicants talk to each other and share their experiences, so they regularly update their selection process and make changes. Also, if you rote-learn answers to specific questions then you may come across as very stilted; if the answer has changed slightly you may find it difficult to answer the new question fully as your mind is already geared to a specific answer.

> Lecturer's tip ... Rather than rote-learn a full answer to a question you think they will ask, try just making a list of key words. It's easier to remember key words and you'll sound more spontaneous when you turn them into sentences on the actual day.

Many of the websites offer messages of reassurance, which is important. Being stressed and nervous can mean that you don't perform to your best ability. It is important that you are realistically prepared and part of that reality check is knowing just how popular nursing is as a career. Nursing programmes receive more applicants than any other university programme, averaging around ten applicants per place. Don't be daunted by this, but see it as a positive challenge. Would you really want to invest in a career that is not valued by others? Also, think how proud you will feel about yourself when you do get a place, knowing just how competitive a process it is.

What are universities looking for?

University selection processes are placing increasing emphasis on what is being described as **values based recruitment** (VBR), which is an approach that is used to select candidates who are able to demonstrate the values, behaviours and attitudes that are deemed important for nursing and align with the values of the NHS Constitution (Health Education England, 2014). VBR has been developed in response to criticisms of nurses and nursing care in the media but particularly in response to recommendations in the Francis Report (2013), which we have discussed in earlier chapters. It would be a good idea to read a summary of the report along with that by the Chief Nurse called *Compassion in Practice* (2012) which details the 6Cs that nurses are required to demonstrate (care, compassion, competence, communication, courage and commitment). Both are now common topics for discussion or questioning at selection days.

Activity 11.1	*Demonstrating the 6Cs*

Think of examples where you have demonstrated each of the 6Cs – care, compassion, communication, competence, courage and commitment.

These do not have to be related to healthcare, e.g. you may have stood up for a friend who was being bullied at school (courage) or volunteered every weekend at a local charity shop (commitment).

As part of your research you may have visited the Nursing and Midwifery Council (NMC) website (**www.nmc-uk.org**). It has a whole section relating to nurse education and very useful information related to student nurses. One of the things that you will find there are the Key Competency Domains, that underpin all nursing programmes so that at the end of the course you are fit and safe to be a registered nurse.

The domains are:

- nursing practice and decision-making (problem-solving skills);
- management, leadership skills and team working;
- communication and interpersonal skills;
- professional values (your personal qualities).

These are important areas to think about now, as many universities are using these domains along with the 6Cs to assess applicants' potential in these areas. In this chapter we will look at how aptitude in these areas can be demonstrated.

Motivation and commitment

Fundamentally, universities want to offer places to applicants who they think are truly committed to becoming a nurse and who have really considered the true impact that doing the course will have on their life. It is not in their interests to have students who drop out.

It is therefore very important that at your selection day you demonstrate a commitment to the field of nursing you have chosen. The fields of nursing are very different, so it is essential that you select the field that is right for you. If you make the wrong choice, it is not always possible to change to another field once you have started your programme.

Activity 11.2 *Demonstrating preparation and understanding*

- Refer back to the information in Chapter 6 about your chosen field and make notes as to why that particular field interests you.
- Reread your personal statement; how did you express your commitment to your chosen field? Do you need to add more for the selection day?
- What resources did you use to make your choice of nursing field? For example, talking to nurses/students representing the field, searching the internet, reading nursing journals, work experience? Make a note of resources used so that you can refer to them at the selection day.

A common question at selection days requires you to show them how you prepared for your interview. By showing that you have made an effort to prepare, you are demonstrating that you are motivated and committed and have the necessary skills to undertake a basic information search.

A good example of poor preparation is when candidates have chosen children's nursing and give as their reason that they like looking after babies. This demonstrates a lack of understanding about children's nursing, as it doesn't reflect the broad age range of children and their families that children's nurses care for.

Challenges in nursing

Like most things in life, nursing has elements that are hugely enjoyable and others that are difficult or challenging. In order to demonstrate that you have made a realistic choice, you need to demonstrate that you have carefully thought about the challenges that you will face both as a student and as a qualified nurse. Again, try and think specifically about your chosen field of nursing.

Activity 11.3   *Challenges in nursing*

- Can you list three situations that all nurses will face that might be unpleasant or difficult?
- Can you list three challenges that would be more specific to the field of nursing that you have chosen?
- For each challenge, consider how you personally would cope. What experience are you drawing on in this consideration?

Sometimes candidates talk at interview about shift patterns or low pay as a challenge in nursing. These are examples that are best avoided, for two reasons. First, they are not specific to nursing; they also don't demonstrate that you are committed to joining a profession that is largely based on shift patterns.

When you think about specific challenges in your chosen field, consider the needs of your patients or clients. Also consider how they and those who are close to them may react to the situation that they find themselves in.

Stress is a very natural response to a challenging situation. Therefore a very common question at interviews is to consider how you deal with stress. Some candidates respond by saying that they never experience stress. Is this realistic? Why might this answer be a problem? Think about stressful situations you have been in: what helped before, during and after? It is better to explain how you cope with stress than to claim you never experience it, as nursing will surely be stressful.

Apart from the reality of having to undertake shift patterns, such as early starts, nights and weekend placements during your training, another reality you will have to consider is the impact of travelling to placements. Unfortunately it is not always possible for universities to send students to placements that are close to their home. You need to demonstrate that you understand and accept this and that you are prepared to be flexible. Flexibility and adaptability are key qualities that universities are looking for and that you should carefully consider and demonstrate during selection.

Again, a common question may be something like, 'How do you think doing this course will change your life?' In applying for nursing it is hoped that you have thought about this already. It is too late once you have started your nursing programme to panic about how you are going to get to your placements, or how you are going to manage financially. These are problems that won't resolve themselves.

Academic challenges

Nursing programmes are roughly a 50/50 split, so you spend half your time learning in university settings and the other half learning in practice situations.

As well as the stressful, challenging situations that you may face in practice, you should consider challenges that you will encounter in an academic setting. In order to do this, you have to consider both yourself and the nature of learning that you will have to undertake to become a nurse – studying whilst undertaking shift hours in practice, for example. You also need to consider the ways that you may be assessed academically. All nursing degree programmes will have at least one formal exam and use a range of other assessment formats, as we discussed in Chapter 5.

Activity 11.4   *Academic challenges*

- If you are aware that numeracy is a weak subject for you, what strategies have you considered that will help you develop your numeracy skills and overcome your fears? How will you improve your skills in this area before you start?
- Another common fear is exams: do you have any examples of strategies that have helped you to be less nervous before exams?
- How will you organise your time to manage the demands of study and assessments?

Personal qualities

Not only do you have to demonstrate that you are academically able and have good communication skills, but also that you have the essential personal qualities we have discussed throughout this book.

You are probably aware of the criticisms of nurses and nursing care that have been discussed in the media. Many of these criticisms stem from concerns that care has been given in ways that are less than compassionate, or even unkind or uncaring. Demonstrating these caring qualities and attributes is extremely important in nursing. It may seem obvious, but without these personal qualities, you cannot be a successful nurse.

Activity 11.5   *Identifying your personal qualities*

- If nurses were caring for someone close to you, what would you consider to be very important that they did for that person?
- Maybe you have had a negative experience of care and that motivated you to come into nursing. Think about that experience: how would you have done things differently?
- In order to demonstrate these caring qualities, what skills do you need? Do you already have any of these skills?

What is important about these activities is that they are encouraging you to think on a deeper level. Rather than coming to an interview and simply saying, 'I am a caring person' or 'I have very good communication skills', you need to think about examples to prove your statements. How do you know that you have good communication skills? It is unlikely that anyone has actually said to you, 'You have very good communication skills'. However, in your personal life, or work or school, people may have said to you 'I can talk to you' or you may have found that people come to you when they have problems because you listen to them well. These are all key elements of good communication skills, so you probably have more positive feedback and useful examples than you thought.

Another important consideration is the difference between personal qualities or attributes and skills. It is important that you understand the difference. Qualities, characteristics and attributes are who you are. Skills are what you do, or how you put these characteristics into practice. Skills can be improved and developed, so enhanced communication skills are one of the key skills that you will develop during your nursing programme.

Very commonly in interviews there is a question about you as a person. It may be phrased something like 'Tell me a bit about yourself; what are you like as a person?' Remember that you should focus all your answers in the context of nursing and the particular demands of the field of nursing you have chosen. For example, if you believe that you are a patient person, you could explore how this quality is important in the context of situations you may expect to encounter. This could be patients who are in pain, depressed or families and relatives who are distressed.

So try and focus on your personal qualities that relate to nursing. Think also of using simple examples to reinforce what you are saying about yourself. Anyone can say that they are kind and caring, but without having examples of how you know you have those qualities, it doesn't really mean a lot.

Being non-judgmental

Another personal attribute that is very important in nursing is the ability not to make judgments about people. This is something that people often say about themselves, but actually they have what we call 'hidden prejudices' that they don't even acknowledge or think about. For example, people often think that being unprejudiced or non-judgmental just means that they are not racist, or can get on with people from different cultures or religions. It actually means much more than that, and applies to all groups of people in society, particularly those who are marginalised. For example, think about the following groups of people and consider how you really think about them.

Activity 11.6   *Exploring your prejudices*

Think about the following groups of people. Be very honest; explore how you feel about them. Have you ever known anyone from these groups?

- drug users;
- the homeless;
- parents who abuse their children;
- people who are HIV-positive;
- gay men or women.

You may come into contact with all these people during your nursing career and you will have to demonstrate a non-judgmental attitude towards them.

Often in interviews there is a question about prejudice, or how you feel about caring for people for whom many people in society have no compassion.

Think of an example of a person that you have befriended – maybe someone who was being bullied because he or she was different. This is a good example to bring to any interview, to show that this is something real for you, something that you have put into practice, even though it may have been difficult for you.

Problem-solving skills

Nursing care is based on the principles of a problem-solving approach. Nurses assess, identify patients' needs and plan care for patients and those for whom they care. How you approach problems is therefore very important. You are probably taking problem-solving approaches every day without realising it. An example of problem solving is how you planned your journey. Did you gather the necessary information together, in order to make the best decision so that you would get to your interview on time? Or did you leave it to the last minute, and rely on other people to get you there on time?

There are many different ways that universities may assess how you approach tasks or problems, for example, group activities or getting you to solve a problem on your own. We will discuss more about these different approaches later in the chapter.

Management, leadership and team working

It is very important that you understand the changing nature of the qualified nurse's role. Nurses already have increasing levels of autonomy and responsibility; this will only increase in the future. Apart from the more obvious roles such as ward managers, nurses manage care in many other ways. Some nurses diagnose and treat those for whom they care. What does this mean in practice? Once they have qualified, nurses may go on to undertake further training, so that they can prescribe medication. You yourself may have visited a clinic that was run by nurses, where all the treatments were given by nurses. We also have specialist nurses that are known as nurse consultants. They are specialists in their chosen field of nursing, so for example we have nurse consultants who are experts and leaders in the care of patients with diabetes, or those with drug and alcohol problems. This may be of interest to you, as you may already be thinking about your future career. It could also be a question at interview, e.g. 'What would you like to be doing in five years' time?'

You may be thinking that you have no experience in being a leader or manager, but actually most people do. Consider Activity 11.7.

As you can see, many activities that are part of everyday life can be used to demonstrate you have these skills. Remember the course will help you to develop them further; you do not have to be perfect at them now, just be able to show that you have the potential.

| Activity 11.7 | *Identifying your leadership and team-working skills* |

- At school were you a prefect, team captain, peer mentor or youth leader?
- Have you ever had to supervise anyone?
- Have you ever been nominated to be a group leader as part of a project or activity?
- Do you play team games or work as part of a team?
- Have you ever been responsible for organising an event for work or friends or family?

The next section will look at the specific approaches to selection that universities may use at your selection day.

The classic interview

The classic interview is one where you will be asked a series of questions by one or more interviewers. If it is just a one-to-one interview, then this will be a member of academic staff who teaches on the nursing programme, usually from the same field as you are applying for. Where there are other members on the interview panel then they could be a qualified nurse who works in one of the areas where students have their practice experiences or a service user who has been prepared for selecting student nurses.

The types of questions that may be asked will vary from university to university but the interviewers will want to know about you as a person as well as your understanding of nursing.

Nursing-focused questions

The following are very common questions:

- Why do you want to be a nurse in your particular field?

- What qualities do you think you need to be a nurse?

- What challenges does a nurse face?

- What do you think is the role of a nurse?

- What do you think makes a good nurse?

- What is the most important quality in a nurse?

- Where does nursing take place?

- Why is teamwork/communication/confidentiality important in nursing?

- What kind of things do you think a nurse does on a typical shift? (likely to be related to your chosen field).

The following types of question are to see what further research you may have undertaken in preparation for your interview:

- Are you aware of any nursing/health topics in the media at the moment?
- What do you know about the course you would be studying here?
- Can you tell me about the 6Cs and give some examples of when you have demonstrated each of them?

Questions about you

- What skills make you suitable for this course?
- What experience do you have that will be valuable to you as a student/nurse?
- What are your strengths and weaknesses?
- What challenges might you face in managing your time and studies on a nursing course?
- Give an example of a stressful situation you were involved in and how you coped.
- How do you deal with criticism/authority?
- What is your greatest achievement and why?
- Why have you chosen this particular university?

Scenarios

You could also be given scenarios at an interview to test your problem-solving and decision-making skills as well as to help the interviewers gain an insight into how you might respond to difficult or challenging situations. Some examples are:

- If you had a large amount of money to spend on healthcare, what would you spend it on and why?
- You have had a bad day and at the end of the shift you have to deal with the death of a patient, and the relatives are angry with you. Who would you speak to about this or seek support from?
- What would you do if the relatives of a patient were becoming increasingly aggressive or verbally abusive towards you?

Video interview

Some universities have used video interviews. These are short videos of children or service users with a learning disability asking a question which you are required to answer as though you are talking to them. It allows them to see how you respond to these particular clients. For example:

Will I be able to bring all my toys into hospital with me?

While you may feel foolish talking to a video (and the university staff will understand that), this gives them an insight into how you can adapt your communication skills for different clients and your ability to demonstrate respect and empathy.

Group discussions or interviews

Group discussions and interviews may be used alongside a traditional interview or be the only selection method used. Usually you will be seated in a circle with other candidates, with one or more interviewers sitting outside the circle making notes on how each candidate performs.

The group discussion

A group discussion usually focuses on a specific topic. This may have been given to you in advance so that you can prepare or you may not know what the topic is until the day.

The types of topic may be:

- current health initiatives;
- how you would invest x million pounds into the NHS;
- how you would manage a child who was refusing treatment;
- what nursing can do to change the bad press it receives.

Important points to remember in group discussions are the following:

- You are being observed on your communication skills, so consider how you relate to others in the group. Do try and make efforts to encourage and support others in the group, even if you don't agree with their opinions.
- You are being observed on your ability to logically and rationally express your views and opinions. Mention any evidence which supports what you are saying, for example the Francis Report (2013).
- You are being observed on your ability to develop solutions and solve problems, so in the discussion suggest solutions to problems, not just criticisms.

The group interview

The group interview is one where a group of students are seated together, usually in a circle, and given questions, which they each answer in turn. They may give you a practice question first. The questions used will likely be similar to the nursing-focused ones we identified earlier in the section on the classic interview. This approach can be quite nerve-wracking, especially if you are last and you cannot think of anything else to say. Rather than say that, consider which of the answers already given you like best, list them and say why.

Preparing for group interviews/discussions

The first thing you need to consider in preparing for successful participation is: what do you think they are looking for? Group discussions can assess your knowledge of a given topic but also assess many different skills and personal attributes. For example:

- Communication skills: never forget that communication skills are not just about talking; listening is equally important. Think about ways that you can show that you are an active listener in the group, even when you are not speaking (e.g. eye contact and nodding). Think about your body language and facial expression.

- Non-judgmental approach: topics for discussion are often controversial; they want to see how you react to other people's ideas and opinions that may be very different from your own. Don't be afraid to challenge people in the group, particularly if you believe that they are being judgmental or offensive. Be very careful how you challenge; think carefully about how you would challenge anyone, without appearing threatening or aggressive.

- Develop *informed opinions*: if you contribute something to the group discussion you need to be sure that your opinion has validity, is based on evidence and is not just your biased opinion.

- Confidence: participating in group discussions can be very intimidating if you are shy. It is essential to overcome shyness and gain confidence in order to become a successful nurse. Remember that nurses are patients' advocates; they stand up for people and protect the vulnerable. Start now.

Group tasks

A group task may be additional to one of the other methods discussed or the only method used. Groups are usually of around four to six and you will be posed one or more questions or given a scenario that may be related to an ethical issue or a more general problem that needs resolving. You will have a set time to complete the task set and university staff will observe how you interact and manage the task.

Again, this may be looking at similar qualities and skills to the group discussions and interviews, but there are additional aspects. Group tasks may also assess the two NMC domains of decision making and leadership and team working.

- Decision making: often the task involves making difficult challenging decisions. Here you may be being assessed on your ethical or moral decision-making skills. For example, you may have to choose which individuals should live or survive amongst a group of people or how the country should manage the increasing obesity problem. Think carefully about the decision-making process. Are you showing a logical, rational approach to making decisions, or are you showing your hidden prejudices? Do be mindful that any task will have time limits, so you may also be assessed on your time management. Even if you are not the leader, be the person who keeps an eye on the time.

- Leadership and team working: you may get the opportunity to be the group leader – don't be afraid to volunteer. Remember a good group leader brings out the best in the team and is inclusive. Look out for the shy, quiet people in the group; give them a chance to be involved. If you are not the group leader think about how you interact with others, listening to them and acknowledging what they say.

Multiple mini-interviews

This approach to selection is well established in medical schools, but is relatively new to nurse selection and is particularly focused on selecting for the values, behaviours and skills being sought in nursing. Kingston University and St George's, University of London was the first university to use this approach for nursing in the UK. The candidate moves round a series of six stations with a set time at each station where they are asked a question or given a scenario or problem to which they have to respond. These will be similar to the ones we have described earlier in this chapter, but may not always be directly linked with nursing. A key aim is to get you to show how you arrive at an answer or decision by talking through and explaining your thoughts as you go, so pre-prepared answers don't work here. Each station will assess the different attributes and skills the university is looking for in a student nurse. You will have a different person at each station so there is greater fairness in the way you are assessed, as several different people will have made a judgment about you.

Lecturer tip ...

- You may well be given a scenario to act out with a role player as part of a multiple mini-interview. Just remember the principles that they have been introduced to in this chapter. What they are looking for are those that demonstrate they have the key qualities and attributes necessary for nursing, not who is the greatest actor.
- As with any situation where you are under pressure, take your time. You don't have to speak straight away, or come up with an answer immediately. If you have time left over, use it to think back over what you have said and whether there is anything important you have missed out.

Asking questions

Remember that selection is a two-way process. It isn't just you who is under scrutiny – so is the university. Spend time beforehand finding out as much as you can about them and their nursing programme. Draw up a list of questions you can ask on the day. If you find all your questions have been answered by the time you get a chance to ask them, still get out your list and check it and tell the interviewers they have all been answered. That way you are showing that you did prepare for questions.

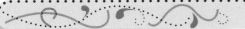

Chapter summary

This chapter has explored the different approaches to student nurse selection and given you the tools needed to reflect and develop the skills and attributes that you have in order to be successful on your selection day. It is a very competitive process so don't be afraid to sell yourself: you need to demonstrate that you have got what it takes to become a great nurse. Also you may enjoy the selection day more than you thought. It is a great opportunity to meet fellow applicants. You may become friends with some of them and share with them the incredible, life-changing journey that is nurse education.

Useful websites

Three websites that are really good for getting up-to-date information on current issues in healthcare and nursing are:

http://nursingstandard.rcnpublishing.co.uk/news-and-opinion

Nursing Standard

www.bbc.co.uk/news/health

BBC Health News

www.nursingtimes.net

Nursing Times

www.prospects.ac.uk/interview_tests.htm

Prospects is a graduate careers website that has lots of tips for interviews and other selection methods.

https://www.assessmentday.co.uk/situational-judgement-test.htm

Examples of situational tests, which although not for nursing students will give you an idea of what to expect.

www.nmc-uk.org/About-us/Our-response-to-the-Francis-Inquiry-Report

NMC response to the Francis Report.

http://www.6cs.england.nhs.uk/pg/dashboard

A website with lots of up-to-date information on the Chief Nurse's 6Cs.

http://hee.nhs.uk/about/nhs-constitution

Provides a link to the NHS Constitution, and lists the values underpinning the NHS Constitution with short videos demonstrating each of them.

Chapter 12
What happens next?

Karen Elcock

Chapter aims

The aim of this chapter is to describe what happens after you have been offered a place or what to do if you are unsuccessful. By the end of this chapter you will be able to:

- identify what you need to do to prepare for starting a nursing programme at university;
- look at the options open to you if you have been unsuccessful in gaining a place at university.

Introduction

Nursing is the most popular course currently applied for at university. Therefore getting past the first stage and receiving an invitation to attend a selection day are major successes. If, following your selection days, you are offered one or more places then you need to consider which one to accept and prepare for the start of an exciting career. If you don't receive any invites to attend a selection day or you are not offered a place after attending one, all is not lost. We will look in this chapter at what happens next for both outcomes.

I have been offered a place

Congratulations! If you are lucky and get more than one offer then you have a set time to accept your chosen place through UCAS. It is more than likely that you have already made your decision, having attended the selection days, but if not, go back to Chapter 7 and look at the areas that we suggested you should consider.

Types of offer

Unconditional offer

There are no conditions attached; you have met all the academic entry requirements and the university is happy to offer you a place. Note, however, that this will still be subject to you gaining occupational health clearance and clearance from the Disclosure and Barring Service (DBS).

Conditional offer

This is usually given when you are awaiting the outcome of exams. The offer is conditional on you achieving the required grades. You usually need to confirm this by 31 August.

How to accept

You have a number of different options when accepting. If you decide that you didn't like any of the universities then you can choose to accept none of the places offered, in which case you would need to reapply through UCAS Extra or clearing (see below). If you have decided to accept a conditional offer then you can also accept an additional offer (as insurance or back-up) in case you do not achieve the required grades in your exams. So there are four possible accept-ances, depending on your offers.

1. Unconditional firm only – you've firmly accepted an unconditional offer. You cannot have an insurance choice.

2. Conditional firm only – you've firmly accepted a conditional offer.

3. Conditional firm + conditional insurance – you've firmly accepted one conditional offer and accepted another conditional offer as an insurance.

4. Conditional firm + unconditional insurance – you've firmly accepted a conditional offer and accepted an unconditional offer as an insurance (**www.ucas.com**).

Once you have accepted an offer you are required to decline all the others (unless one is an insurance offer).

What happens next?

Once you have accepted a place (and achieved the grades required for a conditional offer) then it is all about preparing for your course and life at university. You will receive a letter from UCAS confirming your place and further information from the university. The univer-sity may also invite you to an event to give you a chance to meet your future colleagues on the course and receive an update and advice about starting there. There are key areas to consider:

*   finances;
*   accommodation;
*   travel;
*   pre-reading;
*   the vital luxuries.

Finances

You will need to apply for your NHS bursary; the university will give you information on this. Do remember that you will need to plan for your first month at university before your bursary cheque arrives. You will inevitably have expenses to pay, for example on travel, food and drink, for which you need to plan. It is a good idea in the first few days to eat in the university restaurant or cafe so that you can find out where they are and how much they cost, but more importantly, so that you can mix and socialise with other people in your group. Eating and drinking with other students are great ways of making friends. After the first week you may decide to bring in food and even a flask for your hot drinks to save money.

Accommodation

If you are going to be living away from home, the university can advise you about accommodation, whether in halls of residence or private rentals. If you opt for private rental, check whether the rent covers gas and electricity, water and insurance and that it is secure and within easy access of the university campus. Will you need to pay a deposit, and if so, how much will it be?

> *Student tip* ... The sooner you start looking the more likely you are to get decent accommodation that is close to the university.

Travel

We have discussed this in Chapters 2 and 7, so do look at these chapters again. Once you have your accommodation confirmed, start finding out the best routes to get to and from the university and the costs involved; then ensure you have enough money to cover this for the first month.

Pre-reading

You may want to buy a few books for the course, but it is advisable to wait as the university may organise a book exhibition or will give you reading lists and recommendations after you start. It is also advisable when you start the programme to spend some time looking in the library at the recommended books so that you can choose ones which match your reading style. If you buy books before you start they may not be the right ones or suitable for the course. It is worth looking on websites to see if anyone is selling any second-hand books; you can often find some real bargains. At the end of the course students sometimes sell off their books, so it is worth keeping an eye on notice boards in the university for any adverts. If you want to do some preparatory reading and the university does not provide a reading list in advance, then refreshing your understanding of anatomy and physiology is a very good place to start.

The vital luxuries

Although once seen as luxuries, these items are now almost essential to student life.

- A mobile phone – many universities now use text messaging to keep in touch with students. If you have a smartphone you can access your library, e-mails and the university virtual learning environment, so you can get in some extra study while travelling to and from university.

- A laptop or PC – vital for assignments and literature searches. The universities will have PCs in their libraries that you can use, but that limits how much work you can do at home.

- TV and TV licence – we all need downtime.

- Less essential but really useful are tablets that you can use to take notes in class and access the internet via the university intranet.

Lecturer tip ... It is always useful to reflect on selection day experiences, even when there has been a positive outcome. Did you get 100% on your numeracy and literacy tests? If not, can you improve in these areas? Were any aspects of the selection process difficult for you? None of us are perfect, but evidence shows that the students at university who are most successful are those who can self-evaluate and work on improving the areas in which they are not strong.

I have been unsuccessful

Places for nursing courses fill fast, so it is possible that you were unsuccessful simply because there were no places left. This is more likely to happen if you applied late in the application cycle or to a very popular university or course (the field of child nursing tends to have the greatest competition for places). While it is unlikely to be the case for all your choices, if this is the case you should consider applying to other universities or for a course in a different field of nursing (having thought carefully whether a different field is right for you). If you do decide to change your choice of field, you will need to reconsider your personal statement. If it focuses on a specific field you will need to see if any universities you apply to will accept a revised statement sent separately. In either situation, starting the application process again through UCAS will be different this time, which we will look at later. There are two most likely scenarios if you have been unsuccessful.

1. You have not received any offers to attend a selection event from your university choices.

2. You have attended one or more selection events, but have not received any offers from them.

In both cases the university may inform you as to why you were unsuccessful when it sends the decision. If you don't receive any information you can try contacting the university for feedback on why you weren't successful.

You received no offers to attend a selection event

In this situation your application will have been rejected on the basis of what you have put in your application form and will be for two reasons, which we will look at in turn.

You didn't meet the entry criteria

This shouldn't happen because you should have looked carefully at the entry requirements for each university and if you were unsure you should have discussed your qualifications with those that you were interested in before applying, to ensure you met their requirements.

If you did not meet the entry criteria for your chosen universities, then you need to identify whether your qualifications meet the requirements for any other universities, as these do vary considerably, and you can then apply to those (see section on UCAS Extra, below) or you can wait until the clearing period when entry criteria may be reduced slightly by some universities.

If your qualifications do not meet the entry criteria for any university (even through clearing) then you will need to consider whether you want to study for the appropriate qualifications or reconsider a different course and/or career. The NHS Careers website (**www.nhscareers.nhs.uk**) provides really helpful information on the range of careers in the health service.

Your personal statement did not demonstrate what the university was looking for

Because of the numbers of applicants for nursing, universities cannot interview everyone who meets their entry criteria; therefore, they will shortlist candidates for the selection days by looking at their personal statement.

Activity 12.1	*Reviewing your personal statement*

Take another look at your personal statement and the guidance in Chapter 7. If you can, get someone whose opinion you value to do the same. Be critical and ask yourself:

- Does it show interest in the field I am applying for?
- Have I linked personal interests, hobbies, work or voluntary experience to the skills and attributes required for a nurse?
- Are there any spelling mistakes or grammatical errors?

Note how it could be improved.

The UCAS website (**www.ucas.ac.uk**) provides guidance on writing a personal statement, so look there as well. If you decide to reapply elsewhere in the same academic year you cannot change your personal statement, but you can contact other universities you apply to later to ask if they will accept a revised one sent straight to them.

You have not received any offers after attending a selection event

If you are unsuccessful having attended one or more selection days this may be because you did not pass the numeracy or literacy test (if they had them) or weren't successful at the interview or group discussion.

If you do not pass your numeracy or literacy test you are told on the day, so someone from the university should have given you advice as to how you can improve these skills. Some further education colleges also run classes to improve numeracy and literacy.

If you were unsuccessful at the interview phase, then you need to take time out and reflect on how it went and be honest with yourself. The most common reasons for deciding that a candidate is not suitable are:

- no insight as to what nursing is or what nurses do;
- no understanding of the field applied for;
- failed to demonstrate the attributes required, e.g.:
  - communication skills;
  - team-working skills;
  - being non-judgmental.

Talk to colleagues who know you and ask for their honest feedback; reread the earlier chapters in this book and consider how you can prepare better for future interviews.

Applying through UCAS Extra

UCAS Extra is used when you have used all five choices on your application and have received no offers (or rejected all offers given). You can apply for another course through UCAS Extra between February and July but this time only for one course at a time. If you accept an offer you cannot continue trying for other courses, but if you don't get an offer or choose to reject any offers you can keep reapplying one course at a time until early July. It is also important to note that the university you apply to can see your previous choices so if you have decided to change field they will see that and want to know why. If this approach is not successful or you run out of time then you can always apply through clearing between July and September.

Applying through clearing

Clearing takes place between July and September and is available to students who:

- did not receive any offers;
- did not achieve the grades required for a conditional offer;
- applied after 30 June (these automatically go to clearing);
- declined any offers they received;
- paid the full amount but only applied to one course.

Universities publish their vacancies on the UCAS website so check which ones have vacancies and contact them; try and arrange a visit if you can. Don't automatically accept the first place you get, but do ensure that you keep an eye on the last date for confirming your acceptance.

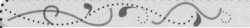

Chapter summary

Going to university is incredibly exciting, but daunting, so ensure you prepare well for it. If you are unsuccessful in your applications then consider how you can make yourself more attractive to universities by gaining additional qualifications or relevant work experience. If all else fails, consider other health and social care courses; the NHS Careers website (**www.nhscareers.nhs.uk**) is a good place to start.

Further reading

Tobin, L (2009) *A Guide to Uni Life: The one stop guide to what university is REALLY like.* Richmond: Trotman Publishing.

A number of these guides to university life are available. This one is a top-seller and looks at finances, health, housing and freshers' week in an easy-to-read format.

Useful websites

www.nus.org.uk

The National Union of Students has useful information to consider before starting university and once you are there.

www.thestudentroom.co.uk/wiki/Before_You_Go_To_University

The Student Room website has lots of advice on what you need to do before you go, plus forums where you can talk to students who will be going to the same university and doing the same course as you.

www.ucas.ac.uk

The UCAS website provides lots of useful guidance on what to do if you are unsuccessful in gaining a place.

https://www.ucas.com/ucas/undergraduate/finance-and-support

The UCAS website also has useful webpages on starting university, including preparation, managing money, student unions and getting support.

Appendix: The Getting into Nursing Timeline

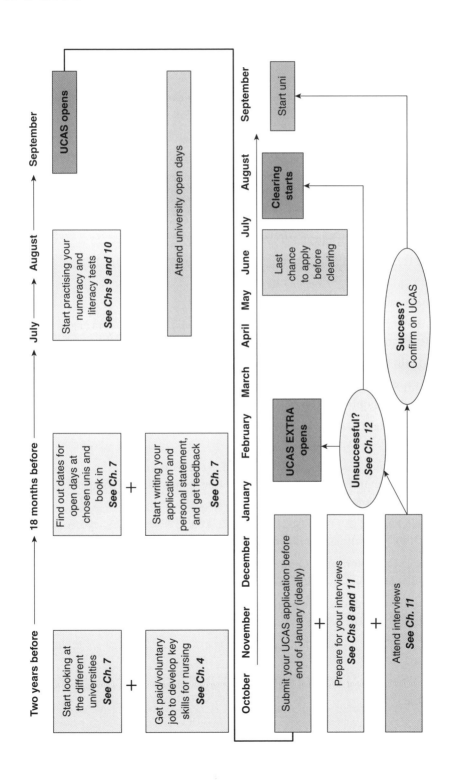

References

Barker, P (2009) *Psychiatric and Mental Health Nursing: The craft of caring*, 2nd edition. Abingdon: Hodder Arnold.

Brady, M (2009) Hospitalized children's views of the good nurse. *Nursing Ethics*, 16: 543–60.

Bridges, J (1990) Literature review on the image of the nurse and the nursing media. *Journal of Advanced Nursing*, 15: 850–4.

Chief Nursing Office and DH Chief Nursing Advisor (2012) *Compassion in Practice*. Available from: www. england.nhs.uk/wp-content/uploads/2012/12/compassion-in-practice.pdf

Department for Education and Skills (2004) *Every Child Matters*. London: DfES.

Department of Health (2006) *Modernising Nursing Careers: Setting the direction*. Available from: www.dh. gov. uk/en/Publicationsandstatistics/Publications/PublicationsPolicyAndGuidance/DH_4138756

Department of Health (2007) *Good Practice in Learning Disability Nursing*. London: Department of Health.

Department of Health (2009) *Nursing Careers Framework Poster*. Available from: www.dh.gov.uk/en/Aboutus/ Chiefprofessionalofficers/Chiefnursingofficer/DH_108368

Department of Health (2010) *Equity and Excellence: Liberating the NHS*. London: Department of Health.

Department of Health (2012) *Liberating the NHS: No decision about me, without me. Government response*. London: Department of Health.

Emerson, E, Hatton, C and Roberson, J (2011) *People with Learning Disabilities in England: 2011*. Durham: Improving Health and Lives. Learning Disabilities Public Health Observatory.

Equality Act (2010) London: Stationery Office.

Francis, R (2013) Report of the Mid Staffordshire NHS Foundation Trust Public Inquiry. Available from: www.midstaffspublicinquiry.com/report

Gates, B (2011) *Learning Disability Nursing: Task and Finish Group Report for the Professional and Advisory Board for Nursing and Midwifery – Department of Health*. Hatfield: University of Hertfordshire.

Gunasekara, I, Pentland, T, Rodgers, T and Patterson, S (2014) What makes an excellent mental health nurse? A pragmatic inquiry initiated and conducted by people with lived experience of service use. *International Journal of Mental Health Nursing*, 23: 101–9.

Health Education England (2014) *Health Education England Values Based Recruitment Framework*. October 2014. Available from: http://hee.nhs.uk/work-programmes/values-based-recruitment/national-vbr-framework

Health and Social Care Information Centre (2009) *Adult Psychiatric Morbidity in England: Results of a household survey*. Available from: www.ic.nhs.uk/pubs/psychiatricmorbidity07

Health and Social Care Information Centre (2014) Accident and Emergency Attendances in England – 2012–13. Available from: www.hscic.gov.uk/catalogue/PUB13464

Henderson, V (1966) *The Nature of Nursing: A definition and its implications for practice and education*. New York: Macmillan.

Lederer, R (2002) *The Bride of Anguished English: A bonanza of bloopers, blunders, botches, and boo-boos*. New York: St Martins Griffin.

Maben, J and Griffiths, P (2008) *Nurses in Society: Starting the debate.* Available from: www.kcl.ac.uk/ schools/ nursing/nnru/reviews/nis.html

NHS Confederation (2012) *Children and Young People's Health and Wellbeing in Changing Times: Shaping the future and improving outcomes.* Available from: www.nhsconfed.org/resources/2012/12/children-and-young-peoples-health-and-wellbeing-in-changing-times

NHS England (2013) Statistics. [Online] Available from: www.england.nhs.uk/statistics

NHS England (2014) *The NHS Constitution.* Available from: http://hee.nhs.uk/about/nhs-constitution

Nursing and Midwifery Council (2009) *Record Keeping: Guidance for nurses and midwives.* London: NMC.

Nursing and Midwifery Council (2010) *Standards for Pre-registration Nursing Education.* London: NMC. Available from: http://standards.nmc-uk.org/PreRegNursing/Pages/Introduction.aspx

Nursing and Midwifery Council (2015) *The Code: Professional standards of practice and behaviour for nurses and midwives.* Available from: http://www.nmc-uk.org/publications/Standards/The-code/Introduction

Office for Disability Issues (2011) *Disability: Equality Act 2010 Guidance: Guidance on matters to be taken into account in determining questions relating to the definition of disability.* Available from: www.gov.uk/government/publications/equality-act-guidance

Office for National Statistics (2005) *Mental Health of Children and Young People in Great Britain.* London: Palgrave Macmillan.

Ooms, A (2011) *Yesterday's Student-Nurses, Today's Nurses: Readiness for work of newly qualified nurses.* Royal College of Nursing Annual International Nursing Research Conference, 16–18 May 2011. Harrogate International Centre, Harrogate, England, UK.

Public Health Nursing Division, Department of Health (2014) *Strengthening the Commitment: One year on.* London: Public Health Division, Department of Health.

Randall, D and Hill, A (2012) Consulting children and young people on what makes a good nurse. *Nursing Children and Young People*, 24(3): 14–19.

Royal College of Nursing (2008) *Healthcare Service Standards in Caring for Neonates, Children and Young People.* London: Royal College of Nursing.

Royal College of Psychiatrists (2010) *No Health without Public Mental Health: The case for action.* London: Royal College of Psychiatrists.

Standing, M (2014) *Clinical Judgement and Decision Making for Nursing Students*, 2nd edition. London: Sage/Learning Matters.

The Scottish Government (2012) *Strengthening the Commitment: The report on the UK modernising learning disabilities nursing review.* Edinburgh: The Scottish Government.

Thomas, B (2014) *Vision and strategy: The nursing contribution to the health and well-being of people with learning disabilities.* Available from: www.england.nhs.uk/wp-content/uploads/2013/12/LD6Cs.pdf

Index